HOW TO STOP SMOKING IN 50 DAYS

ISBN 1-57532-181-5

For information:

Press-TIGE Publishing
291 Main Street
Catskill, NY 12414
http://presstigebooks.com
Presstige9@aol.com

First Press-TIGE Edition 2000
Cover and book design: Drawing Board Studios

Printed in the United States of America

HOW TO STOP SMOKING IN 50 DAYS

BY

HUMBLER ACTS

Press-TIGE Publishing
Catskill, NY

TO DREAM: PERCHANCE TO BE.

CHAPTER ONE

You, as a smoker, have a problem. You, as a smoker, also have an opportunity. If you approach this problem of smoking with a certain attitude, perhaps you will begin to see what the opportunity is that you have. Right now, the word 'opportunity' might sound sort of far-fetched. After all, opportunities have a certain glow about them. They are interesting, wealth-building, important additions to our life. How could smoking be something like that? Well, after a few pages into this 'problem' of yours, perhaps you will see what the 'opportunity' might be.

Have you ever heard people say, "If THAT had not happened to me, I would never have GOTTEN TO WHERE I AM NOW . . ." And when they say 'THAT,' it's always understood that 'THAT' was something awful. 'THAT' was something which, under normal understanding, would be considered bad luck, a rotten roll of the dice . . . 'THAT' was something no one in his right mind would have wished for. And yet, there they were, saying, 'If it wasn't for THAT, I would never be where I am now.'

So let us begin by being grateful for our predicament. Let us give thanks for it and say to ourself that we are glad we are a smoker and that we have this problem. For out of this problem will come something extraordinary. Yet practically speaking, how shall we start?

Becoming Detached

It's challenging at first, and it's never going to be what you might call satisfying, but the first thing we do is LOVE THE HABIT OF SMOKING. Now that's probably a big change from where we are right now. We know we get 'something' out of smoking, but we are probably at a point in our life where we also find ourself hating the whole thing. Either because of health considerations, others' condemnation, our own spiritual dismay with the habit, or countless other reasons, we are down on ourself for smoking. Nevertheless, psychologically, what does this do? It gets us tied up in knots and puts one part of ourself against another. Then we go back and forth. We argue, cajole, threaten, punish . . . over and over . . . as each day passes.

We want to become a bit sly with ourself. We do not want to love the habit genuinely but at least refrain from beating up on ourself because of the habit. We want to make friends.

So now we're saying with as much emphasis as possible: I LOVE MY HABIT OF SMOKING. As we reach for a cigarette or whatever it is, we observe ourself and try to relax with the habit. I LOVE YOU may be said as we find ourself engaged in the whole system of smoking. Whatever resistance we encounter, we should love. We begin to practice civility with ourself. We may smile at the absurdity of it, wondering if we are not possibly a bit ridiculous. Still, let us remember that every aspect of ourself, from top to bottom, should be loved. Every morning holds the image of a person looking in the mirror as the cleaning preparation takes place, saying I LOVE YOU – ALL YOUR PARTS. We need this sort of thing; we need to create a certain friendliness with all of ourself. For we are out to change a habit that is quite complex, and so interrelated with all of ourself, that we have to start with a fresh attitude. We can no longer rely on the bullying, fear-imbedded techniques of old.

We can often use these old techniques for temporary results. In all fairness to ourself, what we often get is not really a 'clean' result, but what is called a 'result where one thing vanishes and another thing begins.' We swap one habit for another. We may not even see the 'new' habit but our friends might. We're acting differently, they might say. That temper that we never had is now quite rough. That impatience that was not part of our armor is prominent now. Also the absent-mindedness, which we never suffered, is a big problem now. Yes, we need to love all of ourself . . . then, when change comes, it will be beneficial.

CHAPTER TWO

The habit of smoking, no doubt, has a long and possibly beneficial history. We know of people who used it to overcome fatigue, fear and many other debilitating moments; and for the efficacy of tobacco in specific moments, we might pay our respects. The image of the peace-pipe being smoked by individuals cementing a kind of spiritual togetherness is also quite moving. Nevertheless, we have not used smoking for those purposes. We have used it beyond its efficacy into the realm of being destructive. We are not prudent users of tobacco. It is time for us to recognize that we are abusing a 'ritual' so that it has to 'go.' But how? How can we make it 'go?' Particularly since 'it' doesn't want to 'go.'

This is where the opportunity is going to take place. With this habit, we have an opportunity to find out more about ourself than most mortals would dare find. We are going to find out more about ourself BECAUSE WE HAVE NO OTHER CHOICE. The guy who doesn't HAVE TO DO THIS isn't going to, because he can get by without this work. We find ourself in this situation. We may find out things that will help us not only get rid of smoking, but go on to many other interests and ideas. This may continue to such an extent that we will look back at ourself and gasp in amazement at what we have achieved.

What we are looking for is a method, something that will take us out of our usual 'sizing up of ourself.' We've all been through that and have said things like,

'I cannot quit . . . I dare not quit . . . I am afraid to quit . . . It won't work. . . ." It's all been said. When we start again with this sort of thing, let us try to reverse ourself. Let us be silently at rest. Let us not keep up the 'racket within.' There has to be a better way.

This so-called way needs to address all of ourself, as well. We, as human beings, are quite manifold. We are not just who we think we are, but who we feel we are, and who we are 'as we move,' and who we are 'instinctively,' 'sexually.' And what about who we are 'on a higher level,' both emotionally and intellectually? We are like the days of the week, sevenfold. Each of those folds needs work and each fold has some input into our smoking. Each gets something out of it and perhaps each loses something from it, as well.

Smoking is not just a habit, it is a commitment that somehow has evolved within ourself. Somewhere we found ourself 'in the dynamics of smoking' where all of our parts got hooked. We are not harmonious with this habit, but we are in some kind of conjunctiveness with all our parts. True, one part—for example a Higher Thinking or Higher Emotional Part—might bemoan the situation, but it has made do with it. It has adjusted to the perversity by creating within itself something that makes it 'okay.' Perhaps it's a rationalization, perhaps another behavior, that nurtures it a bit more than need be.

All speculation, except for the obvious fact that all of us hold together in some way, although we punish ourself with this problem.

If we grasp our situation in terms of seven parts, or folds, of ourself, dealing with our smoking in seven separate ways, we may begin to see that the way out is to begin paying attention to 'their' real needs in the face of this smoking of ours.

We have, therefore, to contact them individually in some way.

Let us call these parts CENTERS, since there is more to each of them than just a part. There is great energy and intelligence and skill in each of these CENTERS. They are truly the majestic workhorses of our being.

CHAPTER THREE

Probably, there is a little resistance, which we all experience, going on right now within ourself over the introduction of the SEVEN CENTERS as a tool for dealing with smoking. As this resistance stirs within us, smile. Accept it, bless and be grateful for it and relax with it.

Everything awaits our own experience in these matters. Only we ourself will ultimately see what we are about with these CENTERS. Let us be calm by allowing ourself to explore. We are nowhere but at the entrance to a 'cave,' newly introduced, which has on the side something written that we cannot yet make out. It's just too dim, at this point, to see what the words say. We aren't sure about the guide and we are not sure what's inside. Yet no one is rushing. It isn't particularly ominous where we stand, and we are a bit curious . . . so let's go cautiously.

Let us write down in our mind's eye, the following SEVEN CENTERS:

1. The Instinctive Center
2. The Sexual Center
3. The Moving Center
4. The Emotional Center
5. The Thinking Center
6. The Higher Emotional Center
7. The Higher Thinking Center

Let us assign each of these SEVEN CENTERS to a day of the week:

MONDAY	The Instinctive Center
TUESDAY	The Sexual Center
WEDNESDAY	The Moving Center
THURSDAY	The Emotional Center
FRIDAY	The Thinking Center
SATURDAY	The Higher Emotional Center
SUNDAY	The Higher Thinking Center

Now, step back a moment and take a deep breath or two. Let's pause and perhaps review this idea. We really aren't that surprised by the idea that smoking is complex, that smoking could well engulf all of our being, all of our parts. That really should not surprise us too much, for if we have ever thought about the phenomenon of smoking, it has probably confused us greatly. After all, we are, to some degree, intelligent, we are people who carry on with our day-to-day responsibilities, and we probably make commitments to others and KEEP THESE COMMITMENTS. No big deal, really. We probably make promises to people every day and, by and large, we KEEP THEM.

Yet the chances are when it comes to our smoking, we have been slightly mystified with its power over us. We really find it hard to be who we are and yet be so buffeted by this behavior of ours. That is why for the most part, we need to take a total view of ourself. We need to address the whole of ourself. For it is then, that perhaps we will shed light on something that will spell a beginning to keeping ourself from smoking.

That is why we should allow for working on this problem in a new way. A way that will offer us the chance for change.

These SEVEN CENTERS may have actual places in ourself and they may not. It is not truly important to try to point to where we think a particular CENTER might be. We are dealing with an idea, a kind of psychology of our humanity, and we only need to consider the possible existence of these CENTERS for something magical to occur.

Now, we ought to make some promises to ourself. We need to have some idea what we are trying to accomplish. Our goal is to KEEP OURSELF FROM SMOKING. In all fairness, this goal may pale as we find ourself replacing this habit with myriads of new experiences. We ought to promise ourself that if we make the effort necessary, we stand to develop a very new approach to our lives.

We have accepted the 'possibility that these centers exist,' and now we need an introduction to a new way of working with them.

We could, of course, start researching what each of these centers is, and look for all sorts of speculative doctrine that has been written on them. That is not going to be our approach. The one thing we are committed to is FINDING OUT WHAT IS GOING TO WORK FOR US. The problem with that goal is that we have a very difficult time reaching it when we approach it by way of 'other people's knowledge.'

CHAPTER FOUR

'Other People's Knowledge' is often difficult to apply when it comes to eliminating our habit of smoking. It is true that many things that work for others should work for us as well, and perhaps they eventually will. Yet there is a point where we need to find out some bit of information about ourself before change takes place.

Perhaps someone mentions an idea that seems proper enough, but when we hear the idea we don't often react positively. Maybe we cannot quite 'buy' the idea. Yes, it sounds good, but something isn't taking when we hear it.

It often seems that no one is able to give us the right set of signals to proceed with our KEEPING OURSELF FROM SMOKING PROGRAM.

Knowledge that others have can only help us when we can somehow 'verify' its truth in those areas that mean something to us. The great challenge of life is attempting to discover what it is that is important to us. Once we can discover what is important, we can begin to see HOW TO KEEP OURSELF FROM SMOKING.

There is one area of ourself where we can begin to find out what is important to ourself. It is an area that most people have neglected, because we are, for the most part, able to exist with other people's knowledge. We are not constrained to survive very often on our own wits. But occasionally someone is in such a bind, and finds this resource quite by accident, or this resource finds them. They find it is a resource they never really took very seriously before.

In fact, there is a kind of prejudice against this resource that has become part of our materialistic heritage. It's often portrayed as a kind of darkness, chaos, misery and turpitude. Occasionally someone pays tribute to it and, of course, history and religion are replete with examples of someone's reliance on this resource.

Let us again pause for a moment and recognize that we are in search of something that will help us. We are not after some get-rich-quick scheme, nor are we bent on finding some secret that is going to give us power over others. We are certain about one thing only . . . We would like to begin to learn HOW TO KEEP OURSELF FROM SMOKING.

We have admitted to some degree that other methods have not worked for us. Or, if they have, we have not sustained them. We are willing to concede our desire TO KEEP OURSELF FROM SMOKING is very great. We would truly love to achieve this goal but, so far, nothing has been available that we have been able to wholeheartedly endorse. So we are at a point where we are willing to consider something new. True, we are not quick to get involved in far-out things, and we are suspicious of pie-in-the-sky pronouncements. Nevertheless, we might give an ear to something that we can attempt without any dislocation of our pride or sensitivity.

The challenge here is to our 'openness.' Can we look at something that is so simple, so basic, with fresh eyes? Can we suppress the impulse to smile or snicker, or if we do, accept it as a kind of protective reaction against the unknown?

The irony of our situation is that we have only to begin finding out pertinent things about ourself for our habit to be assailable from the vantage point of liberation.

A little light is all we need. And it may not take much to get it.

CHAPTER FIVE

What we are about to examine is the phenomenon of dreams. We are all human beings and we all have dreams. Some may say they have few, some may say they have many. Nevertheless, all agree that dreams are something they have experienced. We really know very little about them. There is a kind of difference about them that is hard to describe and there is a directness about them that is often quite startling. We seem captivated by them. We may have read a lot about dreams, or very little, but most of us would agree that, viewed over a long time, there is something about them that is truly strange. It is almost as if some agency regulates them, some very different force. The very existence of such a happening almost amazes us. What can we do with them? Are they just there, or is there something that we can say that would allow us to refer to them in some way?

When we start our car at our 'power command,' it does start. When we flip a light switch, we have light. We begin to become accustomed to such satisfactions in our present world. We may even grow accustomed to people answering our calls over various matters and responding in a way that suits us. If we are the people being called to, we know if we do what is expected, according to some previously agreed method, we will probably be rewarded or paid. Life takes on a certain orderliness in most of these situations.

On the other hand, we are all beaten about by the randomness of things in life. We observe illness, health, good and bad luck, prosperity and poverty often with a sense of puzzlement. How does it work? Why does it go to one and not the other, and then away from the one who had it, and to the one who hadn't . . . ?

Therefore, we cannot really depend on much. We can try to hope, but we can never guarantee to ourself or anyone else that things will be a certain way.

Dealing with dreams is much the same. Often there is nothing really startling to report. Occasionally, fortune seems to smile and reveal the most unbelievable thing. It might be an idea that we have never contemplated as being pertinent to ourself, it might be an activity that suddenly makes sense as something in which we should participate. Sometimes it might be an insight into a relationship we have or don't have with someone—something is there that is truly wondrous.

So our labors suddenly seem worthwhile, as harvesters of dreams. When we least expect it, along comes something that makes the days before, that gave us nothing, seem okay.

Dreams may be a kind of valve for our consciousness. We exist in a certain manner and dreams seem to comment often, not always directly, often subtly, about our particular existence. We may, at times, be told quite explicitly about something we are doing. Still, knowing how to take it is difficult. Is it the truth, and what we are living the lie? Perhaps, but with dreams a definite interpretation is never easy. It all blends in with the rest of ourself. It may say one thing one day and another thing another day, and both may be true. The one thing that may be so, is that dreams fill a certain void in our regular conscious lives. We need them, these dreams, whether we take them seriously or not.

What we are going to try to do is make friends with them. They are part of our being and the sooner they know, whatever their basis, that we want to be friends, that we are no longer going to treat them as unwelcome guests in our house, the quicker we can cultivate some sort of rapport with them.

CHAPTER SIX

We have discussed the idea that we are made up of seven parts, or centers, and we have called them The Instinctive Center, The Sexual Center, The Moving Center, The Emotional Center, The Thinking Center, The Higher Emotional Center and The Higher Thinking Center. We have also discussed the idea of assigning each center to a particular day of the week, starting with Monday and ending Sunday. Now we are going to explore the idea of using whatever dreams we have the night before the particular day and center we are going to work on as a kind of RESOURCE for our work.

We are going to try to enlist whatever help there might be from dreams. Dreams can help us to think and feel, and perhaps, act in new ways that might help us discover for ourself HOW TO KEEP OURSELF FROM SMOKING.

The application of dreams to a particular problem is not new. It might be as old as human consciousness, as we understand it. Many cultures have used this idea and flourished with it. Many individuals in cultures have had to use this idea as a very central means to surviving on their own. Some cultures have introduced the idea to their young as THE METHOD for surviving.

All we are doing is taking an idea and applying it to a modern predicament—that of smoking—and perhaps taking into account the idea that we are made up of many parts instead of just one solid being.

Our society has many comforts to it, many attractions; there is an endless stream of stimuli that keeps us on the road to being the same. The chance of outside influences suddenly redirecting us to something new is very remote. We may get interested in some new fad, but for it to hold our attention for a long enough time is very difficult.

So we need to try to devise a system that is strong enough to coalesce ourself into a new discipline. Still, we need to start sort of cautiously. We are not going to discover much for a while, because we need to get used to the way it works, or might work, before we can expect results.

We have questions, fears and we are impatient. All we need to enlist ourself to do is continue with a little attention.

We are not going to interpret dreams the way we might have heard people do, or the way we may have tried in the past. We are going to treat dreams as a kind of 'experience' given to us and all we are going to do is record them. There are not going to be any secret words or hidden ideas or difficult methods. We do not need any background for this work. We only have to want to see if something is dreamed that has some bearing on our life, upon which we can understand better HOW TO KEEP OURSELF FROM SMOKING.

If we happen to be proficient in some method of dream interpretation, whatever that might be, perhaps we can continue with it and accomplish something as well. The whole emphasis is going to be on taking dreams as they present themselves. If they are picturesque and very foreign, we are going to try to present ourself as experiencing this picturesqueness and foreignness. If there is a pleasing, neat advisory statement about something until now unthought of, we are going to pay attention to it, memorize and repeat it during that particular day.

We are not going to be intimidated by dreams, or at least if we are, not take our intimidation seriously. We are going to give ourself credit for being a proud member of the human race and endowed with this phenomenal gift of dreaming.

Perhaps we will falter and that is okay. We are all prone to do that. We still have to live our life and the promise that something may come out of this effort should keep us trying. At these times we have only to remind ourself that we are intent on learning HOW TO KEEP OURSELF FROM SMOKING. We ought to render some sort of oath taking upon ourself that we will work each day toward this goal. By maintaining some kind of consistency, we will find the odds of achieving our goal greatly enhanced.

CHAPTER SEVEN

We need to prepare ourself with several things. During the period when we are in bed and resting, we are going to be writing down our dreams. We need to have some writing instrument and some notebook, or 3 x 5 cards, scotch-taped together. If we share a bed, we might want to find a little penlight and pen combination that would allow us to write without having to turn on a light.

Whatever is comfortable for us is acceptable. Perhaps we can even train ourself to write without a light. Of course, if we want to try recording our dreams with a tape recorder, perhaps this is fine also.

Getting ready each night is also going to be a challenge. We will start Sunday night, for instance, and try to give a few moments' thought to the idea that we will be dreaming about something relating to the INSTINCTIVE CENTER. In that way, when we awaken Monday morning we hope to have something that will allow us to begin our work.

Once we have some sort of information, no matter what, we can try to spend a few moments making it more legible. The jottings we do at night or in the early hours of the morning might be a bit hard to read. We can help ourself by rewriting, or at least going over what we have written and putting it into some clear script.

We allow a great latitude for what we are going to do with this material. By reading it over and aloud, we can try to project ourself into what is going on. If it's some sort of action or physical setting, we can try to relive the feelings that might have occurred in the dream. If it is some sort of admonition, or insight, we can try to commit it to memory and make it a part of our day.

After a while, we may desire to keep some insights on a card. We can then review them when we have a spare moment or two.

It may also become clear to us that a certain trend occurs in one or more of the centers. Perhaps one center seems to have—or at least have as we are applying information on a daily basis toward it—a certain validity that really impresses us. Perhaps we can put all of those thoughts on a special card.

There are no limits to what we can probably do with this method of applying our dreams to the various centers as we have allocated them to the days of the week. There is only the beginning and the desire to work.

One thing that may become clear to us as we continue with this program is how important repetition (rereading, resaying, rethinking) of our dreams is. Often it might take a half-dozen times before something so simple and so basic suddenly imparts a meaning to us. We should never prejudge the value of a dream as we are writing it down and say, 'This is worthless.' Perhaps it seems that way, but often that which seems so worthless becomes quite meaningful as we review it.

Often we don't seem to have any strength, consciousness, or desire to try to write down our dreams. Often, when we awaken, we can recall we had a dream, but we cannot put words to it. It happens and there is nothing to do but look forward to the next day. There are plenty of days and a multitude of information, so that we never have to mind a miss or two.

Let us try to get started now. We are going to work

with the days of the week, the Seven Centers, and a few ideas that may help us begin. The important thing is to find our own ideas, because only then do we have a chance to strengthen our resolve to keep ourself from smoking.

The key to our success in this venture is to learn more about ourself, what we are interested in, what we really want to become, what thoughts we really want to think, and what feelings to feel. We are going to set sail for new areas that we already inhabit, but about which we hardly know anything.

Let us enjoy this quest. It is probably as exciting as we would ever 'dream.'

DAY ONE—MONDAY

For becoming more aware of HOW TO KEEP MYSELF FROM SMOKING—

Today I will work on my *Instinctive Center* with material from the following dreams:

We are at last beginning to record our dreams. It was Sunday night, and before we went to sleep we prepared a kind of promise to ourself that went as follows:

"For becoming more aware of HOW TO KEEP MYSELF FROM SMOKING, tomorrow, Monday, I will work on my *Instinctive Center* with material from the following dreams . . ."

We put this promise on the top of a notebook or on one of several 3 x 5 index cards, scotch-taped together. Then we put whatever we were using on top of a clipboard so we had support against the pressure of any writing we might do during the night.

Now what happened between then and when we awakened in the morning? Perhaps nothing and perhaps we awakened several hours after we went to sleep and wrote down a dream. Perhaps we went all the way through the night into the early hours of the morning and awakened with a vivid dream, but only remembered a small portion of it. At precisely when we were to arise, with the alarm blaring, we got up and wearily made a couple of word notes that meant nothing to us at the time.

All of the above might have happened, or none of it, but for most of us at some point, something will happen and we can probably record a dream or two.

What can we expect at the beginning? We may find RESISTANCE expressed somehow. We might bear in mind that for the Instinctive Center that first night may show a kind of resentment. Issues might be expressed where we see a kind of, 'Well, you really are making things worse!' or 'You're going to be sued!' There might be a sensation of heat, as if something is too hot for comfort.

We have to remember that although the Instinctive Center is a true marvel of effectiveness and physical achievement, it is also addicted to smoking. If addiction could talk, we can well imagine what it might say. It is not going to raise the white flag of surrender too quickly.

Still, in the background we might be daring. We may want this NO SMOKING ALLOWED to come into effect and that is something for which we should be grateful—that we are willing to take a risk. We should be patient with our dreams. The Centers are being worked on and perhaps what is being shown is a combination of what they see now and what some sort of consciousness envisions.

What we don't want to do is get too concerned with meaning. Perhaps there may not be any, as far as we can see; and perhaps there may be some, but it won't take us far. What may help, in particular, is for us to repeat over and over what we dream, trying to experience what we can with as much of our being as possible.

DAY TWO—TUESDAY

For becoming more aware of HOW TO KEEP MYSELF FROM SMOKING—

Today I will work on my *Sexual Center* with material from the following dreams:

A days passes fast and we scarcely finish one day of work on our dreams than another night is upon us. It is time to construct another set of cards. Have we done this? We need to remind ourself that this is no small task that we are attempting. We should decide that we shall exercise all the will we can to achieve what we desperately want and what others desperately want for us: TO KEEP OURSELF FROM SMOKING.

Notice the tie-in between wanting to stop smoking or wanting to keep ourself from smoking AND being able to work with our dreams. Perhaps it looks silly—like a washing machine tied to a refrigerator, but it is necessary.

What did we learn when we wrote out our dreams from Monday night and early Tuesday morning? Did we see any linkage? Do we get any sort of feeling that we have always been 'away,' so we have never had to deal with something?

Perhaps when we started smoking, the Sexual Center filed along with the activity, or perhaps some consideration of 'sexual formality' occurred as we smoked. It was the thing to do and we were at the age when it seemed part of the rites of being with others, part of the ceremony. If we begin to process that sort of thing, engage in feeling how we got sucked in, we will begin to see the reality of 'original smoking.'

We learned the gestures of smoking. It related to the hands making certain movements, pushing something into our mouth and moving the upper part of our body as well. All a little odd if we really observe it, but definitely necessary if we are going to sell others on the fact that we can do it.

Did the Sexual Center have any talent when it came to smoking, when we first started? No, it was probably only an adventurer. At an early age, we probably thought whatever the Sexual Center did was something we should invest in, and probably did for the most part.

But we are older now. We can recognize a silly gesture when we see it.

We need to tell ourself constantly that as far as getting something from our dreams, we are going to— but it will be like learning a new language. At first it doesn't make sense and it seems impossible that what we are hearing really has a basis in meaning. How do we know we are not being duped? We can only keep on, patiently urging ourself to go through the motions of preparing ourself for each night's dreams; and when we awaken, to strive to get something out of these dreams and to go through the day, sneaking as much attention as we can and proffering it to them.

DAY THREE—WEDNESDAY

For becoming more aware of HOW TO KEEP MYSELF FROM SMOKING—

Today I will work on my *Moving Center* with material from the following dreams:

Every word we dream may prove important as we strive to find some clue about what direction our life needs to take to KEEP OURSELF FROM SMOKING. No one is going to give us the secret. Perhaps we can find stimulation from others' suggestions, but to find THE THING from them that is going to work is unlikely for the long term.

There is much psychology involved in what we are trying to do. To frighten ourself into submitting to a STOP on our smoking doesn't seem to work for most of us. Somehow we can handle the moments of terror, thinking about what might be in store for us, until a change in attention flows over to something else. Soon, we are blissfully smoking, or at least indulging in some thoughtless diversion. That may be the way we are as a human being, and nothing can be done except to know that this is part of our makeup.

As we dream, we may find ourself fantasizing that something big is going to happen and sensing a bit of skepticism that it will. This is part of the beginning awareness of our situation. These are truths to a certain point. Not ultimate, but they are truths as we see ourself currently.

We may also have a dream of something that we wouldn't normally indulge in, like chocolate sauce over vanilla ice cream. Perhaps that is something we might love to indulge in, but wouldn't because of the high calories involved. Let's indulge, if we can, if we dream it. Let us reward ourself initially for even considering the proposition that we will learn HOW TO KEEP OURSELF FROM SMOKING.

We might even have a dream where someone close to us expresses envy. That is an encouraging word. If we have such a dream, we should use it, saying to ourself, 'I envy you.' Why would that person envy us? Perhaps they too have a problem with smoking . . . and here we are attempting to achieve some sort of mastery over it ourself. So if we have such a dream, let us make it part of our day today. Carry it around and say it repeatedly. These are the building blocks for our new structure.

Perhaps, too, we experience some sort of singing, or music, something declaiming a kind of victory over tyranny. As a smoker, do we have any doubt about what this tyranny might be? Suppose, for example, it's some marching song, something from a musical or even a National Anthem of some country. We are told what the song or anthem is, but we do not know the words. This is an instance where we need to try to follow up on this 'gift.' Something is being given to us. We need to follow it up, pursue it, and be able to use it for further reinforcement.

As an example, suppose we hear in our dream The French National Anthem (the Marseillaise) in the background and we think someone might be singing the words. We don't know French and we don't even know the translated English words. Perhaps we could run it down, call a reference department at a library, or the French Consul, or a friend who knows French. Suppose we chase down the words and we come up with the following: (Wouldn't we stand amazed at what we are witnessing?)

'Let's get going, children of the fatherland,
The day of glory has arrived.
The bloody standard of tyranny has been raised
against us,
The bloody standard of tyranny has been raised.
Do you hear in these fields the ferocious soldiers
roaring?
They are coming all the way into our arms to cut the
throats of our sons, our companions.
To arms, citizens!
Form your battalions,
Let us march, let us march!'

If we dream such a dream, and really follow up on what has been indicated, we may experience a kind of moving revelation that is a personal triumph over our adversary—smoking. We could perhaps even make this National Anthem and its translated English words a stirring reminder of what we want to accomplish. Perhaps we can share this sort of revelation, but probably it will not mean as much to others.

The possibility exists that as we uncover our dreams for this day, we find ourself expressing the thought, which might even be expressed in our dreams: I FEEL BETTER. Yes, hopefully we should . . . we will feel better when we start KEEPING OURSELF FROM SMOKING. It would do no harm, with that in mind, to say, "I feel better."

For this day, we may find other thoughts in our dreams. We may find, for instance, mention of going to a movie. Again, this could be another reward to grant ourself. The more we condition ourself to rewards for EVEN THINKING or WANTING to know HOW TO KEEP OURSELF FROM SMOKING, the better chance we have of coming up with something vital for our success.

DAY FOUR—THURSDAY

For becoming more aware of HOW TO KEEP MYSELF FROM SMOKING—

Today I will work on my *Emotional Center* with material from the following dreams:

With this day, we start to get into a realm that might be a bit uncomfortable. We might have a dream where we take someone some place, but only stay a few minutes. We are anxious to get on with something else. This is the kind of dream that expresses impatience over dealing with the smoking problem. We don't want to stick around and get acquainted with it. Perhaps in our dream we don't introduce ourself to the people. We are a little tight-lipped. We don't have to interpret such a dream to understand that somewhere within ourself we don't want to treat this matter in any depth.

Suppose we were to construct a kind of conversation between our *smoking habit* and our *Emotional Center*. Suppose it went something like this:

> (We are introducing them.) "Fellows, we would like you to meet each other. S.H., this is E.C.; E.C., this is S.H. Now fellows, we'd like you to sort of get acquainted. We know you have a lot in common and we know that deep down S.H. is carrying part of the ball for E.C., and we suspect E.C. is frightened with S.H. Nevertheless, let's look at it this way. We all want to live in peace. Perhaps, S.H. could change his tune if E.C. started dealing with things differently. We don't really know how, that is really for you two fellows to decide. But shake hands and look each other in the eye, and have a sense of fair play about whatever you decide . . ."

Now this sort of relationship between these two forces might get us to see things differently. If nothing else, it is an exercise that might bring out something about which we have never thought.

We should always be on the lookout for signs of new activities. An immense amount of good can come from some form of exercise, and perhaps the

Emotional Center declares something unexpectedly for us. We might, as an example, see someone riding very professionally on a bicycle in a dream, coasting and looking very fit. Perhaps this would be an enjoyable thing to do. Maybe it seems absolutely impractical for us to look into riding such a bicycle, but we can always harbor the image and replay it, if we cannot do the real thing. If such an activity strikes a receptive chord, perhaps it will get us on a course of action we would never have thought about with our regular consciousness.

We can exist quite nicely with other people's knowledge, going from the cradle to the grave, but if we want to KEEP OURSELF FROM SMOKING, we often need to dig deep within our own self. It is in doing this exercise that we actively promote our own ideas.

DAY FIVE—FRIDAY

For becoming more aware of HOW TO KEEP MYSELF FROM SMOKING—

Today I will work on my *Thinking Center* with material from the following dreams:

We have been moving alone quite nicely. We are already five days into the first week and we are now experiencing a kind of 'surprise' that we have been engaged in smoking. We may have had some dreams for this day that reflect a kind of "What is this strange dog doing on the upstairs porch? How did he get in here, anyway?"

The thing is, for some of us, our Thinking Center probably had no input into the habit of smoking. We just got into it with no real consideration about what we were doing.

Therefore, a kind of shock now pervades our dreams that can show us that we want quite clearly to 'get rid of this strange dog.' We want to walk it to the front door of our house, where we might discover that the front door was left open. We were just not aware of this before. Now we want to rectify the situation and march this intruder out.

We may also have a dream where someone we know only so casually is living in the same building in which we live. Again, the question: What is he doing here? We didn't know he lived in this building. Sure we didn't because our Thinking Center was never conscious, never really conscious in a truth-conscious way, that we had been smoking.

Again, this same fellow who we didn't know was living in our building, may also start telling us about things that he says we did, but about which we really have no recollection. Again, this habit of smoking never really got permission from the Thinking Center.

We may, of course, find a different trend in our dreams. We can feel certain that at this stage of our work, we are starting to find a different sort of awareness. It is an awareness we have never permitted ourself to feel. We are not getting specific things to do yet, but we are letting in some light. We are starting to take some responsibility for our habit, or at least we are resenting the fact that we have it.

That is a start. We might, at this point, begin helping ourself to experience our dreams more, if we start saying them aloud, drilling them into our waking consciousness. We can rewrite the dream or even type it and carry it around, glancing at it whenever we find ourself with a few spare minutes. As a result, we will find an awareness coming to us that is not so much a literal interpretation as a kind of sensing experience.

Beware of word-for-word interpretations. Beware of dictionary assistance. Read, recite, repeat and repeat. It is a new language and it belongs to us in a very personal way.

DAY SIX—SATURDAY

For becoming more aware of HOW TO KEEP MYSELF FROM SMOKING—

Today I will work on my *Higher Emotional Center* with material from the following dreams:

We might be skeptical about what sort of 'difference' our dreams will contain as we get into the Higher Emotional Center. Perhaps we will not see any difference and perhaps we will notice something that is different. The point for us now might be just to go along with an open mind and a willingness to let things happen. In this way we can gain whatever insight occurs without much internal thinking. We are after knowledge that will work for us and whether it comes from one night or another really is not too important.

What have we discovered in our dreams for this day? What did we dream Friday night that we are going to be working on today?

Let us say we really have a weird one. Perhaps we see something where instead of being the one in charge of a situation, we are the victim. In a very vivid, and perhaps shocking fashion, we are the one who is getting screwed. If we reflect on what smoking really is, we may suddenly sit up and realize that instead of the one *doing* the smoking, we are the one *getting* smoked.

We might have a kind of dream where there is the realization that so much time is being wasted, has been wasted, in some non-functioning enterprise. We may rue the expense involved as well. The dream might deal with people supposedly working on something, but who really are not. Often the picture given is quite pertinent to whatever we do in life, whatever our business or professional concerns might be.

The key to our understanding is always to bring the dream back to what we are trying to do: Become more aware of HOW TO KEEP OURSELF FROM SMOKING. As we review our dreams and repeat what they have to say, it is hoped that we will begin to find ourself genuinely ruing our smoking situation. It has to come genuinely and without pretense. We have to endure a private grief and indignation until we find some way to KEEP OURSELF FROM SMOKING.

We may finally, on the sixth day of our first week, find a hundred dollar bill and two ones on our desk, or something that is a pleasant surprise. "Who put them there?," we might ask. We have only to go back again to what we are trying to become aware of, to realize that when we keep ourself from smoking, it's like finding money.

Nevertheless, whether or not we can verbalize this realization, is not as critical as sensing the surprise, and actively engaging in the experience. Becoming mentally pleased with an interpretation of a dream can often dissipate the overall effect of that dream. We do not want to be only intellectually stimulated. We want all of ourself to know what we are about. It is only then that we will truly know what we have to do, and be ready to do it.

DAY SEVEN—SUNDAY

For becoming more aware of HOW TO KEEP MYSELF FROM SMOKING—

Today I will work on my *Higher Thinking Center* with material from the following dreams:

We need to be prepared in this work that we are presently doing to experience the imaginative, clever, often preposterous scenes of our dreams. There can be a range of humor that often allows us no reaction other than to sit back and smile the smile of someone being confronted with a superior wit. That we can put this wit to some useful purpose, in our case to become more aware of HOW TO KEEP OURSELF FROM SMOKING, makes the experience more beneficial.

Further, we should be prepared for all sorts of controversial subjects. We may be comfortable with all sorts of sexuality, or we may be quite modest and Victorian. Nevertheless, we might all find ourself portrayed in ways that we would not want our friends, neighbors or relatives to know about. Whatever the deep-seated reason for all this material, it is all very helpful in getting our attention and causing us to see something in an entirely different way. It is with such insights that new processes begin in our thinking and feeling which may produce a new way of being.

Let us suppose that after retiring for the night, a heterosexual male dreams of seeing his employee, a heterosexual and heavy smoker as well, taking a shower in a black slip. In the dream, the dreamer is giving this man some woman's casual clothes to wear—after some dressy affair he was at—thinking he might want to change. When his employee gets in the shower, his hair is cropped short and he asks the dreamer to pull the curtain around one side of the stall so he has privacy.

Now, reflecting on this dream, we may or may not come up with the term 'drag queen.' This is a perfect description of the heavy smoking that we are addicted to doing and one that we would never have thought of in a million years. That we are experiencing this dream, ought to leave us, if we are a heterosexual, with an uneasy feeling about our habit. We may not say the words, but we would be a bit amazed with the picture. We would not want to say, in light of what we are trying to do—KEEPING OURSELF FROM SMOKING—that everything is just fine. We are forced to see that what we want is a 'stall' and some time for 'privacy.'

Likewise, others who have a different sexual orientation, might dream something entirely different. The point is, that whatever we are or think we are, we are going to be shocked if we allow it. It is in such shocks that we begin to see shades of the truth. Again, we should review the dream and try to regain the moment when we are in the dream, so that everything becomes an experience.

In this seventh day, where we are at the end of the first week, we might also dream about sweets or a treat that we don't want to eat yet. Often, people take sweets or a treat when they commit themselves to not smoking, but here we might see that we are not ready to make the commitment. At least we are putting the sweets somewhere in the hall table at the entrance to our old house, perhaps the same house where we found that stray dog several nights ago.

Are we beginning to experience some success?

We are not supposed to be too successful too soon. After all, we have just gotten into this pursuit. We can only press on with our willingness and good humor in tow.

Perhaps we are going to have more fun than we think . . .

DAY EIGHT—MONDAY

For becoming more aware of HOW TO KEEP MYSELF FROM SMOKING—

Today I will work on my *Instinctive Center* with material from the following dreams:

We may have started getting into the swing of recording our dreams last week and then something came up. Perhaps we had to make a trip or had already planned a vacation. We then found that we really could not focus on this work once we got away from our regular bed and surroundings. So be it. We may always find such interruptions and nothing can be done but to try to get back on track.

It might be that the first night of this second week does not yield much in the way of dreams. So many opportunities are available in this program, a night or two of lost dreams means nothing. It is our intention that is crucial. If we are sincere or trying to be sincere with ourself, we will eventually find just what we are looking for. It will then seem as if everything could not have worked out better.

Let us say that we have one very small dream on this second attempt to 'hear from' the Instinctive Center. We write it down, repeat it often and, although we really can not quite understand it, there does seem to be a message involved. Often we have to ride it out and see if in the writing exercise there is some connection between what we are trying to learn and what we ultimately need to do. There is this mystery about expressing ourself that seems to reside in the fact that we cannot understand a thing until we begin to work on it actively. The meaning is not there immediately, but gradually comes into focus as we work on expressing what the words say.

Writers talk about this often: They have a book that slowly starts to take form and yet they are the witnesses of its creation rather than the creators. Perhaps we can start to use this 'blind faith approach' in expressing our dreams. Not in an intellectual-effete way that springs from what we think other people have told us, but in a quiescent-intuitive way. We need not be afraid of making a fool of ourself, because we are on our own. So we try to express what we cannot fathom without so expressing it. We are like spiders who start to spin a web not knowing from where the thread comes, but only acting instinctively on the impulse that a web is necessary for survival.

Perhaps we have a dream where we are getting prices on something from one place and then quoting them to another place, with some markup. We are not sure what the markup should be, since we are probably going to quote the 'premier supplier' of the very thing we are trying to sell. A very ridiculous situation. Who would dare do such a thing? After all, would we buy something at, say, a very small retail store, mark it up and then try to sell it to, say, Wal-Mart? Would the buyer at Wal-Mart not say to us, "What in the world do you think you're doing? Do you really believe you can get me interested in such a ridiculous proposition? Do you not see that I can 'buy and sell' the place that you get this price from? Your markup is so out of line with what I sell this for that I am almost laughing at your naivete while you insult me with your arrogance. You are wasting my time! Good bye!"

As we look back on this attempt at expressing our dream, we can see a link between how-not-to-be-in-business and how we often try to sell ourself on things that part of us laughs at and rejects. We cannot interest that part in such a nonprofessional way. Either we have to come up with something really spectacular, that the main buyer is going to see some self-interest in, or else we are going to be laughed out of his office.

We, therefore, can see that the Instinctive Center is such a buyer. We cannot meekly approach it with some fanciful idea that will get its attention; and this is all right to understand. We are up against toughness personified. It is only going to get involved when it sees something truly astonishing. Well, since we know our customer, we should be able to prepare ourself for the ultimate sale. It is thinking that we can sell when we really cannot that leaves most attempts at selling on the rocks.

DAY NINE—TUESDAY

For becoming more aware of HOW TO KEEP MYSELF FROM SMOKING—

Today I will work on my *Sexual Center* with material from the following dreams:

Occasionally we find ourself having a dream that clearly is preparing us for some direct help. The idea that we have to work extra hard to interpret dreams is often blown away by the directness of some dreams. It is almost as if they are quite capable of saying something very clearly when the time comes for such clarity.

In such an instance, perhaps we have such a dream as follows:

> We are at some meeting where there is planning for some event. We mention how when we see some huge thing happening and see someone talking about it, and they are photographed simultaneously, it never seems they make a connection. The person is small and the event is big and there is no connection. Then someone mentions the value of getting guidance of some sort through dreams. *They will even tell you what to want to do*, or something like that. They talk about having another meeting to discuss what they need.

We may have some difficulty with parts of this dream, but we have to be impressed with the directness that most of it has. The fact that it occurs in the Sexual Center makes it even more impressive. Let us pause to think how incredible the link is between a single sperm, an egg and the conception of such a high level being as a human being. How many of us have not thought: How can there be a connection between the smallness of the act and the hugeness of its consequences? Likewise, we may further ponder that for many of us the power of our spirit is so incredibly small compared to the immensity of our tobacco addiction.

We do not need to stretch on and on if we do not feel like it. The point that weighs most markedly is when we saturate our thoughts with the words in the dream and try to sense the meaning for us as individuals. Each of us may come away from similar dreams with different impressions. Still, for all of us the meaning will have an influence on our eventual ability to KEEP OURSELF FROM SMOKING.

We simply do not have to worry or fret about what is going to show up for us to be able to follow. We need only to put in the time and effort. We have an inborn sense of what is right and wrong for us in life that dreams help us understand. While we may discuss our plight on one level or another, and find ourself unable to reach any definite form of action, we will have a dream with an entirely new perspective that leaves us in utter amazement.

We do need guidance and we do need to know what to want to do. We give ourself too much pressure when we try to decide our fate or allow others to decide it for us, without having recourse to what our dreams hold up to us.

We need to know that whatever our feelings, no matter how hopeless they may seem, there is a connection between keeping our sense of self and KEEPING OURSELF FREE FROM SMOKING.

DAY TEN—WEDNESDAY

For becoming more aware of HOW TO KEEP MYSELF FROM SMOKING—

Today I will work on my *Moving Center* with material from the following dreams:

As we try to fall asleep at night, we may have a hard time focusing on our little statement above. We need to work on the idea of committing ourself to a repetition of the statement. For example, 'For becoming more aware of HOW TO KEEP MYSELF FROM SMOKING, tomorrow I will work on my *Moving Center* with material from the following dreams' should be said over and over. It is this dedication to the dream process that will yield results far more quickly than a haphazard statement as we lay down to sleep—and then nothing further.

There can be despair if we awaken dreamless at 4:00 or so, and we know we need to be up at 6:00. We might easily feel that it is over as far as any more dreaming. It is never over. We can dream up to the last minute before we awaken; we could awaken at 5:30 without anything, doze off and have a particularly meaningful dream in the last thirty minutes or so of sleep.

We should never give up with the repetition of the statement. We need to try to make it part of ourself, not just some dumb thing we are trying to do. We need to try to focus on each word, saying it to ourself with a certain emphasis on the syllables—and determined concentration. From having little affinity to the statement as a whole, we may become quite comfortable and convinced of its value for us.

We are at Day Ten and perhaps we have a dream as follows:

> We are sitting at a desk in an office and find ourself using a phone that has an exposed wire section. It is also a rotary dial type of phone. Someone comes and puts his hat on a hook above our desk. We are the boss here but do not seem to have any of the appurtenances of bosshood. We fear someone at the desk is going to bring us a bunch of our present paperwork. We would love to be able to jump on stuff and process it immediately. We have been trying to reach someone on the phone but can not make the connection.

We should have little trouble linking our smoking situation to our dream situation of being a boss in name only. We are beginning to exhibit a certain awareness that things are not as they should be. We would love to be able to jump on stuff and process it immediately. Also, we would love to be able to do what we need to do to keep ourself from smoking. So far we have not been able to, but we seem to be trying to reach someone . . .

One interesting thing about doing what we are trying to do is that we may come up with interesting turns of expression that describe some problem we have in general as well as in relation to our smoking habit. In the above dream, our saying "We would love to be able to jump on stuff and process it immediately" might reflect a common problem we have, and recognize, but have never phrased quite like we have here.

What is advised is that we start making little cards with such sayings on them that we can repeat as we go through the day. Not only are these sayings our knowledge of ourself, but they give us a particular attentiveness about working on ourself. They can begin to build up within ourself a certain new form of esteem, one that says, 'Yes, I know my faults, and I can deal with them as I live each day . . .'

This built-in determination results from our becoming aware that our faults are the very thing we need for development at the start. Indeed, there is nothing we need to fear about ourself, if we are sincere in trying to deal with our faults in a positive way. We are beginning to see, hopefully, that learning HOW TO KEEP OURSELF FROM SMOKING might be only the tip of our newfound knowledge.

DAY ELEVEN—THURSDAY

For becoming more aware of HOW TO KEEP MYSELF FROM SMOKING—

Today I will work on my *Emotional Center* with material from the following dreams:

We may, with even the stoutest of efforts, fail to record any dreams. We must always recognize that we can never dominate the dream center, wherever it is or however it works. Dreams are gifts that come from some unusual source within or around us and we need never think that upon our command we will receive what we want, when we want it. So often, or occasionally, we may come up with nothing reportable.

Or it may happen that we have a dream that talks about 'borrowing.' Along with such a dream, it may occur to us that the night before we had several dreams, but time only permitted us to deal with one of them. Perhaps the thing to do is to borrow the material that we did not deal with and work on it today. In other words, if we need some material, and we did not get it last night, we can borrow some from the night before.

Eventually, information we are looking for, which will show us HOW TO KEEP OURSELF FROM SMOKING, might merge into some kind of whole thing anyway. So let us look and see what we might have dreamed the night before and did not have time to work on:

> There is some fleeting dream about some guy saying it is refreshing to see someone in his area who doesn't drive a Porsche or have some van, and so forth, when it comes to think . . .

We might review this dream a number of times and if we get nothing out of it but a sense that it is reflecting our methodology, as something refreshing, that would be enough. If we further think that perhaps the dream is saying that our methodology is not very professional looking, that should show us that what we are doing is very simple, almost naive, but perhaps quite valuable.

We might have another dream from the night before last that we never got a chance to reflect on:

> We hear that someone is going to take
> their mother and father on a trip.

We would normally look past such a dream and say inaudibly to ourself, ‘So what?’. Yet we are trying to be quite open and ready to receive any sort of help we might get to become more aware of HOW TO KEEP OURSELF FROM SMOKING. Is there, therefore, anything in this dream that might help?

It is precisely here that the refreshing part might become important. One of our parents may be deceased. So “parent” might take on a very subjective theme. Is smoking a power over us the way a parent used to be? Are we powerless as we used to be as children?

Also, if we happen to have such a dream and one of our parents is still alive, perhaps it would be nice, and something we’d never otherwise consider, to take a parent on a little trip. Perhaps such an act might do something special for us and them, which would enhance our life and theirs. It might, in some unknown sort of sequence, bring us closer to KEEPING OURSELF FROM SMOKING.

What we are learning through this work on dreams is how sacred we might become as we seriously consider new ideas as potential sources for our self-improvement. Only we, ourself, as an individual, can say and do what we dare feel and think. No one can arbitrarily conduct our life based on his interpretation. We may look for common clues and patterns, but ultimately we have to live our own life as befits us.

DAY TWELVE—FRIDAY

For becoming more aware of HOW TO KEEP MYSELF FROM SMOKING—

Today I will work on my *Thinking Center* with material from the following dreams:

Without disclosing disruptively vulgar dreams, we need to understand that we might all have them, and benefit tremendously from them, in private. There is a clarity about them that needs recognition. Often, it takes something really crude, really outrageous, to make us look at what we are doing with freshly shocked eyes and ears and maybe even nose.

We have gotten away from our earthiness with much so-called education, breeding and reluctance or fear of facing our human nature. So often, what we dream is not so much an indictment of our lack of conscience as an indictment of our reluctance to use it.

When we were young, we faced this human nature with a sort of glee and friendliness, but now we do not. Of course, many inbred prejudices never go away because we never get beyond them. Dreams use prejudice, among other things, as a helpful way of proving a point. Perhaps, as we grow—which might occur more often if we follow the dream tips provided with some prejudicial reference—we no longer need prejudice to prove a point.

We need not proclaim these dreams publicly to recognize their value. We might find in them some really basic information that will get us moving in the direction of KEEPING OURSELF FROM SMOKING.

On this twelfth night we may still find that we are reporting some already reported themes and a few new ones. One thing we need to be patient with is how this work is progressing. So far we have spent as much time in talking about reacting toward the idea of KEEPING OURSELF FROM SMOKING as we have in witnessing any new ideas or actions that might promote us in that direction. Yet that is the way it might need to go for most or all of us.

We need not think it is a waste of time. Getting the proper motivation often comes after first disclosing to ourself all our objections or doubts or questions. Once the light of day touches all these defenses, then perhaps new material can enter our consciousness.

Maybe we have a dream about doing some exercising or meditating under someone's guidance and when we do it on our own, someone says it is difficult. Here we may be expressing the idea that our program to KEEP OURSELF FROM SMOKING, on our own, might be difficult.

True, it is one thing to be entertained by someone else's efforts and another to start doing the thing ourself. There is nothing wrong with recognizing that perhaps the Thinking Center is putting out such an idea to forestall our efforts from continuing.

At this point, we just don't know how our allies are going to develop. We need to remember that for how-many-years-only-we-ourself-know we have been smoking and polluting our mind. It may not be any wonder that perhaps our mind is not able to give us full support.

It might even happen that one night we get some support and another night we do not. If we just keep on plugging along we will finally reach a consensus where we can really do something totally committed to KEEPING OURSELF FROM SMOKING.

We may have another dream on this twelfth night that goes as follows:

> We are with a group of people and we are going to eat dinner at some fancy place and then find we have to get the table ready. There is a little table where we are going to have to put a big one. We find ourself picking up broken glass and saying to someone, 'We are not going to get this thing together and have to *pay* $50.00 a couple—we'll do *that* for $40.00 a couple!'

Lastly on this twelfth night, perhaps we have a fleeting dream where we see an elderly lady in a store. She is in the store a long time just sort of walking around.

DAY THIRTEEN—SATURDAY

For becoming more aware of HOW TO KEEP MYSELF FROM SMOKING—

Today I will work on my *Higher Emotional Center* with material from the following dreams:

No one can say that KEEPING OURSELF FROM SMOKING is easy and learning or becoming aware of HOW is not easy either. But hopefully, we are going to all look back once we complete our journey and say, "Whatever the pitfalls and the pratfalls, we made it!"

For right now, we are still receiving mixed messages, which truly reflect our ambivalence and indecisiveness. Perhaps we receive one dream where someone is saying the lights are out and it is hard coming out from a side lane, so we had to stay in the main stream of traffic.

On the other hand, maybe we receive a dream showing an acquaintance of ours looking super thin. Starting a program that would get us in that sort of shape might be enjoyable. But then we also have a dream where we are standing at a counter receiving someone's cash for something. We put it away and we do not remember how much is given. We stumble about trying to remember and the buyer waits for us to complete the sale. We keep fumbling around trying to find the money and recall how much change we should give him.

Then, along comes another dream where someone calls a fellow smoker "nice." They turn to us and say, 'But not you.' Our reply is, 'Thank you.'

This night has all sorts of variations, as if we are doing the work of five men. Perhaps we are five men, or women, when it comes to finally being able to KEEP OURSELF FROM SMOKING. Perhaps it really is Seven Centers that will ultimately vote on our joyous transition from smoker to nonsmoker. We are, however, still in the primitive area of KEEPING OURSELF FROM SMOKING.

Take a dream where we might come into a room and start joking about something being spectacular when it is not. Then we really feel like smoking and someone near-and-dear to us gives us a frankfurter out of their sandwich, leaving them with the bread.

We are still perhaps a bit ‘chicken’ about really doing something in the way of change. We are probably more interested in operating our computers than in defining our actions. But being able to recognize our present state is all aprt of the process.

DAY FOURTEEN—SUNDAY

For becoming more aware of HOW TO KEEP MYSELF FROM SMOKING—

Today I will work on my *Higher Thinking Center* with material from the following dreams:

We are now completing two weeks of dream work dedicated to learning HOW TO KEEP OURSELF FROM SMOKING. We probably find the days passing very quickly as far as not having much time to spend on our dreams.

How much time are we spending? How much time do we have to spend? If we spend at least thirty minutes a day, we have a fair chance to make some impact on ourself with our search. If we spend more, all the better. If we are only spending a few minutes a day, looking at our dreams for some revelation, we may be cheating ourself. Often the value of a dream only comes from persistent repetition and experiencing. We are simply not able to get an immediate fix from a dream. At least, we are wiser not to go at it that way. Exceptions occur, but the general rule needs to be to plod along and work at it.

Often, a dream's meaning will not come to our mind, but we get a rhythm or nursery rhyme effect from our dreams. The more we repeat it, the more it has this kind of effect. If someone asks, “What does it mean?,” we can take a stab at it but there is more awareness from parts of ourself that are not literate.

Another thing to bear in mind is how familiarity with the words starts to breed a meaning that is personal for us. If we were to talk about it, we would not feel very confident in explaining the dream. We would wonder about our stability. Still, on our own, we are aware that it is saying something personal and we are grateful for the experience.

Experiencing dreams may be like experiencing forms of art. We might wonder what in the world is going on at first, but over a period of time, something seems to appear. For now, we might still be in that state of mind called despondency over the possibility of losing our habit. Perhaps we have a dream like the following:

> We are at some prestigious foreign university walking around wearing only undergarments. We seem to be slightly infatuated with someone of the opposite sex that we are looking for. We have a cigarette that we take a drag on but it has no tobacco. We seem to do nothing all day. We're getting no mail. We think, 'Maybe we should take a shower' but we do not seem to find our dopp kit. We go into the office, turn and go another way when we see someone in the office.

We may, in some part of ourself, want to change but we have an overwhelming unwillingness to clean house. Perhaps on this night we have a dream like the following:

> We seem to be giving a man money to go to the bank to get change from a cash register. But in the cash register drawer we find all sorts of cut up paper—for

> what we do not know. Possibly it could be for stuffing boxes if we were to send an item through the mail. When we try to pull out handfuls of the stuff and throw it in the wastebasket, a lot of it misses and falls on the floor. What a mess! We seem to think we will just wait for the cleaning man to take care of it.

Or perhaps we have a dream that might be advising us that when we do start to work on this search to know HOW TO KEEP OURSELF FROM SMOKING, we should rely on our own work and not on others:

> Something about a guy asking us about some computer thing. We quickly tell him we do not know. Then he asks a guy next to us, who very confidently seems to produce some sort of formula which, he says, will take care of his problem. He then discusses piracy and how his company has tried to go to court since he knows there's libraries, etc. all over that are using the stuff. We seem to have sat before and eaten—or something.

This then is as far as we may get after two weeks. We need to double our efforts as we go into the third week. We need to be as earnest with ourself as we can, really wanting to find out HOW TO KEEP OURSELF FROM SMOKING.

DAY FIFTEEN—MONDAY

For becoming more aware of HOW TO KEEP MYSELF FROM SMOKING—

Today I will work on my *Instinctive Center* with material from the following dreams:

We have gone through the entire night and early morning with scarcely a note on our dream card. As we lay awake trying to get the last thirty minutes of rest, we find ourself somewhere between dreaming and being fully awake. In this period of thirty minutes we have a couple of unusual words or phrases that come into our mind.

Often, these 'intermediate periods' produce interesting ideas. These ideas have a kind of superior directness that cuts through many difficult dreams.

Perhaps on this morning we have a one-word sort of 'revelation.' The word is DECONGESTION. It is a word we probably never use in our so-called waking existence, but there it is written on our card. Then, between sleep and awakening, a phrase pops into our mind: "You know what you need? . . . is a hook on the door!"

Finally, moments before we finally awaken actively, we experience the phrase *Books and Documentation.*

When we have a moment—after we are out of bed and can spend some energy in reflection—we sense a kind of elation with the word DECONGESTION. For if we have one thing to report about our cigarette smoking, it is the feeling of being congested in the chest. We may have been feeling this more recently than ever, or maybe we experienced it a while back and succeeded in forgetting. Now that we have a tangible word to say to ourself (DECONGESTION), we have to feel that it would be truly wonderful if we could experience DECONGESTION and not CONGESTION.

As we think about this word and what it means, it is almost as if now we are prepared to do anything to achieve this word. Yes, finally we have a word that is almost like a mantra. We can say this word over and over, and it will strengthen something in us toward our goal of KEEPING OURSELF FROM SMOKING. We may have different words and these might appear any time. Such words start to prepare us inwardly for our journey and accomplishment.

We next take some time to reflect on the phrase, "You know what you need? . . . is a hook on the door!" Maybe we are tempted to think that it applies to some current problem we may have with a gate or door. Dreams are interesting that way.

For that matter, intermediate dreams often take something that is quite mundane, something that we are experiencing, however passively, and use it to help with something of greater import. Here, we are trying to get material that will help us become more aware of HOW TO KEEP OURSELF FROM SMOKING. We have the word DECONGESTION, which has given us an idea of how it would be if we did not put so much smoke in our lung area. Is there any connection between that word and the phrase: "You know what you need? . . . is a hook on the door!" . . .

Well, perhaps a connection does exist. We find ourself repeating the phrase, almost as if it is the line of a song, and what comes to us is a kind of advisory—we need to use that word DECONGESTION as a hook on our door. If we really want to experience that word, we would, in effect, be putting a hook on our door: This would prevent us from putting a cigarette to our lips and drawing in smoke through our mouth.

Finally, we look at the phrase *Books & Documentation*. Perhaps we find in this phrase a kind of advisory to search out what really is going on with the congestion in our lungs. There are many books on this subject. Or, we are getting a thought that maybe there will be books for us to look at as we go along on our search. We know books are out there about the problems with smoking, but we have never wanted to bother with them up to this point. Nevertheless, if we have this sort of dream, maybe it means we should be willing—if the right book is made known to us.

As for documentation, maybe it is time to write down, to document, how we really feel as we smoke. How does the smoke feel as it goes into our mouth and lungs? Maybe we need to document such things. And have we ever described other things that go on while we smoke?

DAY SIXTEEN—TUESDAY

For becoming more aware of HOW TO KEEP MYSELF FROM SMOKING—

Today I will work on my *Sexual Center* with material from the following dreams:

One interesting thing about recording dreams is the follow-up that is often required. Take the following dream that we might have on this night:

> There is something about being with a man who seems to be Tom Sawyer at some point in his life. He is an older man now.

As we look at this dream, keep in mind that we are trying to become more aware of HOW TO KEEP OURSELF FROM SMOKING. We also want to understand the dynamics of our Sexual Center. We have to think that the character of Tom Sawyer must be referring to us. It is always natural to assume that a name in a dream, particularly a literary character, is referring to us. Yet do we really remember much about Tom Sawyer? Perhaps we have not thought of this character for years, apart from an incidental literary item that we might have read. He is not part of our conscious waking thoughts, but here he is in our dream. We would like to know more about him. Libraries have reference departments with people manning them who have almost instantaneous reference skills that can help us with this kind of question. For a brief moment or two, we can find out something new and something that our dreams have deemed important for our consideration.

Of course, those of us who have access to the Internet can perhaps call up information from there as well.

Perhaps what we learn about Tom Sawyer makes us feel something about our own youth, when we first started smoking and having sexual experiences. It takes a few moments of reflection to get something from this kind of knowledge. It does not smack us in the face. Slowly and subtly we might get a sense of insight into who we are and who we used to be. For we really are not who we were then and yet, as far as our smoking, we might be thinking we are.

Along with the Tom Sawyer dream, perhaps we also have the following dream:

> There is something about having bought a huge sort of pedestal and we and someone else are trying to push it up a stairwell. The man with us seems to be

> the one with the strength. He stops pushing and it turns and falls over. We remember feeling it is so heavy we too have to let it go. It falls and damages one part of its edge at the tip.

As we experience this damage to the pedestal, there is real distress. A kind of shock that it just could not have happened. It's an awful surprise to see the damage done. We need to relive our dreams over and over during the day in which we are working on them. Often, not trying to figure them out is better until we have gone over them. Sometimes we can cave in to an easy explanation and lose some experiencing, which is probably the most important part of the dream.

The pedestal falling is not what we want to see happen. Yet the nice thing about a dream is that it gives us the experience without inflicting the loss. We do not have to live with this damaged pedestal once we awaken. We can grow from the experience some way, even if we really do not know how. We have an influence upon us that is almost as real as if the fall had actually happened.

And in the same period of this night and early morning, we may record the following dream:

> Also, we seem to be driving a cart up some stairs and people are sort of admiring us, although at one point we can't make the corner on one try.

The experience here is more gratifying, although there is the last moment or two when we can not quite do what we want. Are we getting close to understanding the dynamics of our problem with smoking? Are we at least admitting that something is wrong with us? Something, perhaps, but not everything.

Every night and early morning of dream recording brings us closer and closer to our goal of knowing HOW TO KEEP OURSELF FROM SMOKING. Giving up the fight would be easy and understandable; and when we awaken after a dream that is not particularly pleasant we may experience fear. Yet in the conscious light of morning, we can probably handle ourself with a certain strength and courage that will carry us on.

We may not be having much fun. However, we can be assured that once we have been able to KEEP OURSELF FROM SMOKING, we will be painstakingly different and truly *having* fun.

DAY SEVENTEEN—WEDNESDAY

For becoming more aware of HOW TO KEEP MY-SELF FROM SMOKING—

Today I will work on my *Moving Center* with material from the following dreams:

Perhaps on this night or early morning, we have the following short dream:

> There is some conversation about going on a journey. We are going with some other people. At first it seems we are going to take a bed and maybe even a chair.

There is something sort of bizarre about taking a bed and maybe even a chair as we experience it in the dream. Who could go to that much trouble, much less even have a chance of pulling it off? After all, no one takes a bed and chair . . . But then, as we think about it later, maybe our journey consists in just that: taking a bed as we dream and taking a chair as we work on the dream. There is a feeling of finally, perhaps, getting ready to make some sort of commitment.

If this is so, perhaps it is a good time to reflect on just what material we might have acquired within our last sixteen days of dreaming. Make up a little spread sheet with headings of all the Seven Centers from *Instinctive Center* on the upper left and *Higher Thinking Center* at the far right, and the remaining Centers placed between them. Pull from any of the dream cards pertinent information that we can use for some positive reinforcement as we begin our journey. We will probably find only a few things, but hopefully for us they will be very important things. We may find something like the following:

Under *Instinctive Center*, we have put two items:

DECONGESTION

"You know what you need? . . . is a hook on the door!"

Under *Sexual Center*, we have put one item:

Then someone mentions about the value of getting guidance of some sort through dreams—*they will even tell you what to want to do.*

Under *Moving Center*, we have put four items:

The French National Anthem, in English:
'Let us get going, children of the fatherland.
The day of glory has arrived.
The bloody standard of tyranny has been raised against us,
The bloody standard of tyranny has been raised.

Do you hear in these fields the ferocious soldiers roaring?

They are coming all the way into our arms to cut the throats of our sons, our companions.

To arms, citizens!

Let us march, let us march!'

We envy ourself.

We feel better.

We would love to be able to jump on stuff and process it immediately.

Some of us may have a different result. It is interesting that here we find only the beginning three Centers yielding anything that we can use as positive reinforcement. Hopefully, as we proceed, we may begin to accumulate more knowledge that will ultimately show us HOW TO KEEP OURSELF FROM SMOKING.

DAY EIGHTEEN—THURSDAY

For becoming more aware of HOW TO KEEP MYSELF FROM SMOKING—

Today I will work on my *Emotional Center* with material from the following dreams:

How are we doing? Are we hanging in there? Do we see the subtle thing we are trying to do towards becoming more aware of HOW TO KEEP OURSELF FROM SMOKING? Some of this work is going to be difficult and perhaps it is already difficult to explain. We are inculcating (within) a kind of strategy that is very personal and very effective as we continue. We have no outward proof that what we are doing is going to work.

Nevertheless, what we are doing, or trying to do, is similar to what people do when they listen to very advanced music or view very advanced painting. They are feeding their mind, their brain, with new food that often does not quite sound or seem right at first. The irony in all this is that to grow, we have to experience new things. We cannot grow by doing what we have always done. We have to expose ourselves to new directions, new disciplines. If we are afraid to stretch our mind and heart, we cannot change for the better. True, there is some risk but there is greater risk doing nothing new.

As we go along night after night, we signal to our inner self that we want to work on our dreams and centers. Our primary purpose is to become more aware of HOW TO KEEP OURSELF FROM SMOKING. Perhaps the secondary purpose is for some overall greater appreciation of ourself and our world. To attain these purposes, we have to be patient, hopeful and positive.

On this night, or early morning, perhaps we experience the following dream:

> Some men from the government appear and seem to need something and we take them to find someone near-and-dear to us who is apparently working for us. We find him sitting with a young girl on a tractor and kissing. We reprimand him and tell him after 4:30 he can do that. We then tell him to take the men and find what they need.

Are we at last trying to cooperate with some greater power and urging some rebellious instinct to cooperate likewise? It sounds promising, if nothing else. Following the preceding dream, we may also have another:

> We seem to be lying on our back and with our feet almost planted flat, springing up into a standing position.

Again, this appears promising. It is hard and the fact that we can do it, may show some sort of ability to get back on our feet. An exuberant image, if we think of ourself snapping to attention from a life of inattention to our smoking habit.

Although we put some meaning to these dreams (more as a means of working with the phenomena than out of necessity for its effectiveness), the better way is simply to inundate our thoughts with the words. The whole thing is nothing more than developed repetition. We discipline ourself to keep on with the few sentences that we record every night until a kind of pattern emerges that we can identify with.

We are moving steadily toward something. We may not feel it much but, as sure as we can count on daylight, we can count on some sort of arrival at a new place. It will be at this new place where we can KEEP OURSELF FROM SMOKING.

DAY NINETEEN—FRIDAY

For becoming more aware of HOW TO KEEP MYSELF FROM SMOKING—

Today I will work on my *Thinking Center* with material from the following dreams:

The *Thinking Center* means to be a bit higher up for us than say, the *Emotional Center*. So when we have a dream on behalf of the *Thinking Center* at night or morning, we might want to put a little pressure or attention in our head as we focus on the dream. That might help us get a better sense of what is being said. We are not really out to establish some sort of "Thinking Mode," but it is amazing how a little pressure will give us a new direction. It's almost as if we go from somewhere in our chest to somewhere in our head and discover what thinking is all about.

For those of us who do not perform this little exercise much, we might have the following dream:

> There are people over at some little house where we are and we seem to be busying ourselves with emptying ash trays. As we are doing this someone near-and-dear-to-us talks to a friend asking her if she is interested in some sort of entertainer or music in town. She is not. And then some woman wants to know something for her kid who sits at the table.

We may surmise from this dream that some little house where we are could be the place that is not very big in our lives, the *Thinking Center*. Similarly, the fact that we are busy emptying ash trays may be a kind of thoughtless task that shows that our tolerance for smoking is shrinking. If not yet quitting, at least we are getting rid of the evidence and reminder of the habit.

Perhaps it is stretching, but it may seem to us that smoking and entertainment and music in town seem to go together. It seems as if a kind of wavelength exists that all are on. The fact that our friend says she is not interested is also a good sign. The little kid's mother wants to know something. Could we hazard a guess that it's—"What can I tell my kid, or what would you tell your kid, about smoking?" Is there any one of us who would recommend to anyone's kid the idea of smoking? Wouldn't we all say, "No way! Don't start, and then you won't have to find yourself confronted with all sorts of problems!" Probably we would all agree by now on at least that much.

Although we are not yet KEEPING OURSELF FROM SMOKING, at least we would willingly advise others to KEEP THEMSELVES FROM SMOKING. Being able to say this, at least lets us know we are moving in the right direction. It's really not that we need a fancy new mind, but that we start exercising the one we have and appreciate the fact that it is quite adequate for all our needs.

DAY TWENTY—SATURDAY

For becoming more aware of HOW TO KEEP MYSELF FROM SMOKING—

Today I will work on my *Higher Emotional Center* with material from the following dreams:

With this night, and this center, we experience something that is truly amazing. We may have a dream or two where we see writing on possibly some type of newspaper article, manual or any written format. The thing that is amazing about this dream is that it never seems possible for us to read and remember the entire portion of the writing. It is almost as if it's there, but not yet available for us to partake of. However, there is a subtle hint that sometime we can probably get it all. Perhaps one of our dreams goes as follows:

> Some sort of an ad in a newspaper—
> SPIRITUAL UNIVERSAL.

When we reflect on this short dream, we recall it is on a full page of ads and the phrase 'spiritual universal' is either in one of the ads or as a heading. Hundreds of words, perhaps a thousand, appear on that page and yet all we get is 'SPIRITUAL UNIVERSAL.' Does this have anything to do with our goal to KEEP OURSELF FROM SMOKING?

We see nothing joining the two ideas. We need to reflect on these dreams with a certain trust that somehow whatever we are dreaming allows us to accomplish our primary goal. Reflecting on the term 'spiritual universal' might impart a certain sense of freedom. It is as if our mind-set, whether it is a particular spiritual leader or a general religion, is suddenly allowed to be loosened.

In another society, in another age, perhaps people would have a hard time understanding why people would be happy if they won the lottery or inherited much money. They might wonder, why is there a connection between one thing and another? Perhaps our wondering what might be a connection between 'SPIRITUAL UNIVERSAL' and KEEPING OURSELF FROM SMOKING merely reflects a certain conditioned lack of experience. We may also have another quick dream of the following:

A COLUMN—ARMY GROUP

Again, as we reflect on this dream, we vaguely recall that there is another article in a newspaper and the heading appears to be ARMY GROUP. There is undoubtedly information in this article but we just can not read it, much less remember what it says. We can spend as much time as we have available reflecting on this barest of information versus the most extravagant possibilities for our learning more.

If our *Higher Emotional Center* could combine the discipline and directiveness of the ARMY GROUP with the deeply satisfying meaningfulness of 'SPIRITUAL UNIVERSAL'—and apply it to KEEPING OURSELF FROM SMOKING—we would truly have something. Still, all we need to do is repeat the words and let them sink into our mind. Further, we may dream something like the following on this night:

> We are going through some manual and finally get to where we need to be. We see a note or hear that some guy is with someone else in need, using that particular material.

So again, we have to see that we are not yet given the answer, although we might be getting indications that the answer is near. Lastly, we may have one of those one-sentence dreams that goes as follows:

> You might kick out the bugs.

It is almost as if the dream is saying, "While we are waiting for the answer, we might as well clean house, exterminate, kick out the bugs!" We all have some and, for some of us, bugs and bugbears may be synonymous.

DAY TWENTY-ONE—SUNDAY

For becoming more aware of HOW TO KEEP MYSELF FROM SMOKING—

Today I will work on my *Higher Thinking Center* with material from the following dreams:

Sometimes, when we awaken during the night or early morning—not finding ourself mindful of any dreams we may have and yet feeling some sort of need to express ourself—we may resort to taking hold of our clipboard and night light pen and writing something like the following:

> 'We may think of the struggle as the downside, the unnecessary, but it may be that which is more important, more necessary, than a moment of success.
>
> 'The more we try, the more we find, the more we try, the more we find: it is all an exercise destined to bring us success but success in due time not necessarily according to our wishes.'

We may find it hard to live and believe the words that we write down, but it is always a good practice to let such thoughts register in our mind. Perhaps the truth in them does become at some point part of our presence—for working on what we are presently doing or later for other matters.

After we have fallen asleep again and reawakened, perhaps we find ourself writing down the following short dream:

> If we pressure something, we may omit a few important steps.

No doubt, we are beginning to feel pressure about our becoming more aware of HOW TO KEEP OURSELF FROM SMOKING. Maybe some of us have long ago reached a conclusion about what we need to do and are now doing it full force. Perhaps we are sensing all the successful feeling and thoughts that must undoubtedly accompany such an attainment. We are happy for whomever those people might be. The rest of us are still struggling with many precepts that may be helpful but are not yet the answer. So it is good at such a juncture to reflect on the dream we just had:

> If we pressure something, we may omit a few important steps.

We may not know what those steps are but, if we feel ourself pressuring, it is probably a good indication that there are still a few important steps yet to take. We may also, on this night or early morning of the twenty-first day, have another quick dream as follows:

> Something about giving it all the attention we could.

We think at first that the dream is saying that *we are indeed* giving this work all the attention we can muster. Then we have another dream which goes as follows:

> We say girls are probably like guys. They sit around talking about what they are going to do and then go home and forget about it. Maybe the quietest little guy who no one suspects is getting a lot.

So are we talking to each other now, but going 'home' and forgetting it? Let us resolve, in this new week just coming up, not to forget. Let us resolve to give this work all the attention we can muster.

DAY TWENTY-TWO—MONDAY

For becoming more aware of HOW TO KEEP MYSELF FROM SMOKING—

Today I will work on my *Instinctive Center* with material from the following dreams:

Inching along, in stages, we may wonder what is going on. We have been pursuing this line of reasoning or discipline for a little more than three weeks and perhaps we are still in the dark. We occasionally have a glimpse of some promise or two, but we are not particularly happy with our predicament. This is the kind of journey that is necessary. If others clearly mark the way, there can be no exploration. If there is plenty of light, we can not be on a self-discovery mission.

We are so used to using other people's knowledge. We just do not feel comfortable doing this sort of thing. If we simply persist, despite our feelings of frustration or bouts of ill temper over the pursuit, perhaps we will be victorious. The fact that we have a very definite goal may just keep us going. We sincerely want to be able to KEEP OURSELF FROM SMOKING. With all else either failing or not making a permanent dent on our habit, we elect to pursue this unusual course.

So what do we dream on this particular night or early morning? Perhaps we have a kind of glamorous looking dream that goes something like the following:

> We go with someone near-and-dear-to us to some play and we're a bit late. Some woman converses with someone near-and-dear-to-us and then we go in and go to a window where some dangerous scene is going to take place. There is even a sign saying DANGER or DANGEROUS SCENE.

Everything in this dream is so pretty and neat. We recall the very lovely woman that talks to our partner, and then the scene at the window is quite beautiful. The danger sign seems so muted, although the word is DANGER.

As we reflect upon this dream repeatedly, maybe for some of us a sort of parallel dawns between the glamor and the danger of smoking. We never really think of it that way and we cannot really say we feel this DANGER now, but in some part of us there is the realization that some dangerous scene is going to take place.

Again, inch by inch, things begin to add up. Not according to others' time table, but according to our own. Perhaps we awaken a bit later, with only the following statement of a dream:

> Few things in modern times have had such an impact . . .

"At first we have no idea what this dream refers to, but then we think of other people who have stopped smoking: they often report that all of the things they have accomplished, keeping themselves from smoking ranks way up there. Perhaps the discipline that we are embarking on will have the same impact on our life. The habit of smoking, as we practice it in these modern times, has an impact on us like few other things.

Often, the openness of a dream statement allows it to play around us freely and allows us to do with it as we may. Perhaps the following dream continues with a similar line of reasoning:

> Something about a phrase in Latin that seems to mean from many there is something—and it speaks of something that comes from various parts of society. We think the Indian Nation is mentioned.

Again, maybe a kind of instinctive reflection that smoking is a combination of factors coming from many places. However considered in the past, can we question its consequences today? Later, just before waking, perhaps we have a dream like the following:

> We see a guy—perhaps a little disabled—get on the back of a truck in the bed and crouch. The truck pulls away. We think for a moment the driver isn't aware of the guy, but he evidently is—since he stopped at a spot he wouldn't have stopped at, unless he was waiting for him to get on.

We have a bit of pity in our hearts as we see this poor fellow hitching a ride and yet it might just be that he is getting a lift to some place where he could not go on his own. This is sometimes the mercy contained in a dream.

DAY TWENTY-THREE—TUESDAY

For becoming more aware of HOW TO KEEP MYSELF FROM SMOKING—

Today I will work on my *Sexual Center* with material from the following dreams:

What is it like to wake up every morning, or most mornings, and record dreams that are surprises and filled with an agenda we cannot fathom? A mystery that causes us delight along with our puzzlement? What can we say?

First, are we still working on our goal? Sometimes, we make no apparent connection between the words in the dream and our goal. Are we able to keep going, with faith that occasionally gold will emerge from all this panning? We are still looking for meaning, though we might want to go with the proposition that it is the experiencing of the dream that will give us what we need. (Yet would a little meaning hurt?)

All we can say is that dreams will give us what we need when we need it. Dreams refuse control or twisting by our will. This does not mean that we cannot receive the answer we seek, here HOW TO KEEP OURSELF FROM SMOKING. It is just that we have to endure many things beforehand. It is like the ancient custom of becoming acquainted with someone: it often takes a long time before one can conduct any official business. Therefore, we must endure and practice some patience as we put in time and effort with whatever we are given. Perhaps we have a kind of positive dream that goes as follows:

> It seems we are somewhere and see a converted gambling vessel pull on the river and then turn around. It is moving swiftly. We are very moved to see it and say, 'That's from a familiar city.' Then we walk to the beach area and it is beautiful. The sky is a beautiful color and there is clean, white sand. It looks as if there has been tremendous development.

Anytime we see the word 'development,' we might take heed and have courage. Perhaps something is happening in our lives, something that might just pay off in the achievement of our goal. Following that dream, perhaps we have one, something like the following:

> Something about being somewhere and finishing with something and then hoping one of our near-and-dear-ones will come by and give us a ride. It is starting to drizzle slightly and we begin to wonder how we are going to get a ride. We begin holding up our hands as cars and trucks pass, not really hitchhiking but sort of hoping in the midst of the traffic, there will be a ride—perhaps a cab.

What sort of experience can we get out of this last dream? Can we live through it with some sort of impression? Is it vague no matter how hard we try? There is an earnestness and intensity, an uninhibited gesturing for some sort of help, that we feel as we attempt to relive it. Does this give us anything? We can only say that a desire to get a ride somewhere exists. A kind of eagerness to get from where we are to some place else. That is something, not a lot, but something.

Next, we may dream something that comes totally unexpected:

> We seem to see an article on Gabriel Heater in a tux and realize that when we were children, Walter Winchell was who our parents listened to—"Good evening, Mr. & Mrs. North America and all the ships at sea!" It seemed there were so many voices and discussions coming out of the radio.

To be able to dream such a dream and say it aloud, to be able to dream such a dream and recall a lost part of America's past, not really to know what it says and yet appreciate something about it—this is the gist of work on dreams. Something touches us, prepares us and beyond that we have a hard time saying. Perhaps in some way, it echoes a sea-change in our own life.

Lastly, on a night that might have its fill of dreams, perhaps we have another:

> There is also a dream about seeing new movie houses being built. It seems as if there are going to be four, as if there is one on each side of a big square building. It seems as if they are all connected within the body of a huge square block building.

These are not modern movie theaters with many screens in one area. They are converted movie houses of old that seem to have new faces and much inner togetherness that are old-fashioned in the equipment shown. Just to sense the structure with our mind and gut may give us some new experience that prepares us for something finally useful.

DAY TWENTY-FOUR—WEDNESDAY

For becoming more aware of HOW TO KEEP MYSELF FROM SMOKING—

Today I will work on my *Moving Center* with material from the following dreams:

Sometimes we seem to dream about something that we are occupied with, but the dream seems to use it very differently. Understanding the significance is difficult. It is so close that we find it hard to both focus and try to figure it out. We can get bored with repetition. The answer just might be to accept the disquieting effect of a dream that does not seem to do much. Just accept it and, of course, it might be just the effect that we need in order to progress.

As an example, let us suppose that we have been thinking about a spiral staircase leading to a roof with an enclosure at the top. We dream the following:

> Apparently there is some new guy working for us at our company and we show him or try to show him what we want as far as a spiral stair to the roof. But it gets complicated as we don't seem to find the same elevations leading to the first part of the building. There are different ways of going now. He does say there is some sort of spiral stair already made for about a hundred dollars. We still do not seem

> to get to tell him about the little house we want on top.

What we do believe is that dreams will not play games with us when it is time to talk real talk. There may be much of 'a little bit of this and a little bit of that' in dreams like the above, and we have to accept it. When we are ready, a dream comes, an experience occurs, which makes no bones about the meaning. We couldn't hide from it even if we wanted to. So perhaps what we really have to admit is that we say we want meaning, but then when we really have it, we try to look for some way out. That might be the way we are.

We may also have another dream on this night or early morning as follows:

> There's a dream where someone near-and-dear-to-us comes to see us at some new quarters we have as an office. It's quite frugal looking. It has a modest sort of living room and when we invite this one and another in we wonder about the dimness of the lights. We also notice a bunch of papers on a table, all sorts of games, etc. We couldn't even find a calendar to check something we are referring to—a Mother's Day thing. Then we seem to have to rush away and later come back and are reading about someone in the government who has something to do with dreams of others. There doesn't seem to be much air down there nor much business. It is away from the general operation, we guess. One of the two near-and-dear-to-us has to walk down a long flight of steps to get to it.

Perhaps we are simply being forced to experience a transition—whether it reaches upward or downward. This is part of our gradual discovery of what it will take to KEEP OURSELF FROM SMOKING.

DAY TWENTY-FIVE—THURSDAY

For becoming more aware of HOW TO KEEP MYSELF FROM SMOKING—

Today I will work on my *Emotional Center* with material from the following dreams:

The dream that we experience on this night and early morning is really unique. We never had such an experience and we might have really thought we were ill as we experienced its sensations. All that we write down is the following:

> We have a kind of bitter tasting effect as saliva goes down our throat and wakes us up—as a number of plates are seemingly in our mouth or we swallow the saliva on them.

What we may not record is the actual taste. We may think we have an upset stomach or indigestion. We may think the dream isn't reflecting our smoking habit or dawning impression of the habit's vulgarity. When we awaken and begin thinking about the entire phenomena of awful tasting sensations, we have to wonder suddenly if the taste isn't some simulation of clumps of raw nicotine deposited on our tongue or down our throat. We experience the taste of an acid-like substance that we have occasionally experienced at a much lower intensity when we have had a poor nicotine exposure—more likely with a pipe or cigar than with a cigarette, but nonetheless reminiscent of all three.

So here we are startled at this really alarming turn of events. We may have been thinking that perhaps a breakthrough would come in some kind of burst of understanding, where we would clearly see how we could KEEP OURSELF FROM SMOKING. Now we have this awful lingering sensation that really could affect our smoking without any insight at all except that we do not like doing to ourself in small amounts what we have just experienced in a big amount. Whether such an experience takes or not we will see individually, but we are gradually getting help from each center in ways peculiar to them.

We may ask how does the *Emotional Center* get involved with a dream where we experience such a terrible sensation of raw nicotine? Perhaps what we experience is something like a representation of our feelings, dressed in basic abhorrence of all forms of tobacco. As we have said before, once something needs to be expressed, dreams do not always express it softly. There seems to be 'no-holds-barred' once we are ready to gain an item of understanding.

DAY TWENTY-SIX—FRIDAY

For becoming more aware of HOW TO KEEP MYSELF FROM SMOKING—

Today I will work on my *Thinking Center* with material from the following dreams:

We are nearing the close of the fourth week of night-to-night, day-to-day dream work. We ought to be getting some definite signs of help, though for each of us they may be quite different. What we are seeing here are dreams that we have, but it should not disturb or surprise us if our dreams are quite different. A great phenomenon of dreaming is how individualistic each dream can be. We may all work similarly, even act similarly, but we can dream quite dissimilarly.

What we may dream this night or early morning is nothing more than the following:

> There's a call of our name and we see someone at the door and go over to open it.

That is all we can remember and probably all we are ready to accept. At least there is a feeling of promise or something new. No foreboding, only a willingness to see whoever is there. Perhaps the dream is only to get our attention and allow us some time to see what we have already learned from our work over the last four weeks.

We have already listed what we learned a few weeks ago and now is the time to review those things plus new things we find. Again, this is what we find, but the same format can be used for those of us who find very different items.

Under *Instinctive Center* we put the following items:

DECONGESTION

'You know what you need? . . . is a hook on the door!'

There's . . . a sign saying DANGER or DANGEROUS SCENE.

Few things in modern times have had such an impact.

Under *Sexual Center* we put the following items:

Then someone mentions about the value of getting guidance of some sort through dreams—*they will even tell you what to want to do.*

It looks as if there is tremendous development.

Under *Moving Center* we have the following items:

(The French National Anthem, in English)
'Let's get going, children of the fatherland,
The day of glory has arrived.
The bloody standard of tyranny has been raised against us,
The bloody standard of tyranny has been raised.
Do you hear in these fields the ferocious soldiers roaring?
They are coming all the way into our arms to cut the throats of our sons, our companions.
To arms, citizens!
Form your battalions,
Let us march, let us march!'

We envy ourself.

We feel better.

We would love to be able to jump on stuff and process it immediately.

Under *Emotional Center* we put one item:

A bitter tasting effect as saliva goes down our throat.

Under *Thinking Center* we are putting one item which we may have possibly dreamed earlier and neglected to acknowledge:

Do not look at women.

Under *Higher Emotional Center* we are putting two items:

SPIRITUAL UNIVERSAL.

'You might kick out the bugs.'

Lastly, under *Higher Thinking Center* we are putting the following items:

If we pressure something—we may omit a few important steps.

Something about giving it all the attention we could.

This then is our little bag of personal self-knowledge. We may not value someone else's, but we should find our own quite worthwhile. We may carry this list around with us, pausing to reflect on it during our day. Perhaps when we are waiting on a line to take us to where we are buying something or for another event to take place. A few scattered moments throughout a day may enlist our attention wisely and profitably.

We do not idly pick up this information in someone's book or magazine article. We do it through our own effort and tribulation. Now that we have it, let us put it to work in the only way we can at this point—through thinking it and feeling it. What comes next is not necessarily in our power, but it is within our power to set the next chain of events into some order.

DAY TWENTY-SEVEN—SATURDAY

For becoming more aware of HOW TO KEEP MYSELF FROM SMOKING—

Today I will work on my *Higher Emotional Center* with material from the following dreams:

We have probably all heard stories of explorers who run out of money or time and have to abandon their exploration. Then time elapses and someone else comes along, returns to the spot of the original explorers, and reaches what they could not. It always seems so sad to think that another moment, another day, a week or whatever, and the sought after treasure would have been discovered by the first group.

Perhaps we have a similar problem facing us; and perhaps it is worse. Because if we do not mind our own being who will? Maybe there is some kind of human continuum that passes from generation to generation, but it also might be that we have something within us that is ours. If we do not deal with it, it is lost for good both for us and for what it may do for others.

So working with a sense of seriousness is important. Of course, what we are trying here may not seem THAT serious. We are trying to gain insight that will allow us TO KEEP OURSELF FROM SMOKING. We cannot expect any tremendous gifts for such a pursuit. On the other hand, once we achieve this goal, there may be other more noteworthy things for us.

So what we need to talk about for a few moments, is HOW we approach our dreams in the context of what we are trying to achieve.

First, we are starting with our goal, which is HOW TO KEEP OURSELF FROM SMOKING. This is an idea that should be uppermost in our mind as we get ready for bed, go to sleep, and awaken periodically during the night and early morning. We need to give our attention to this idea. Once we achieve this goal, hopefully we can go on to other things if we choose. However, for these hopefully limited number of weeks, we need to dedicate ourself to HOW TO KEEP OURSELF FROM SMOKING.

Along with this goal, we also need to focus as intently as we can on the various centers that we are dealing with as night passes and the day begins. If it is Friday night, we need to begin focusing on our *Higher Emotional Center* and for all of Saturday, we focus on the *Higher Emotional Center.*

Perhaps it is just not necessary to focus on anything else. Those of us who are spiritually inclined may want to bring in some 'help' from Our Higher Power. Maybe for some it is okay, but some kind of danger can present itself. Our smoking habit is a particularly ugly, dirty thing. We need certain 'tools' to deal with it. Other tools may not be 'earthy enough' to help us. If we are in the garbage business, we do not drive to the 'site' in a passenger car. We use a garbage truck. Sometimes, we enlist our Higher Powers for service where They are perhaps less powerful than our own earthly tools. They can be quite useful in giving us faith, hope and love (and of course, countless other qualities), but we might best affect the actual business of working with our smoking problem, with what we have.

Now, the most important part of our work, after we dream dreams and write them down, is going over them. It is here that we need to try to do something that might seem odd, difficult or even uncomfortable. We need to try to keep in mind as we read our dreams: BOTH our goal of HOW TO KEEP OURSELF FROM SMOKING and the PARTICULAR CENTER with which we are working.

It is this practice that might give us important clues to what we are experiencing and what we are saying. It almost seems as if doing this exercise unlocks the dream and allows us to sense as NO ONE ELSE could tell us just what is going on and what we need to do.

The use of the various centers may seem far-fetched UNTIL we see it work. Then 'common sense' takes a back seat to the phenomenon of experiencing.

DAY TWENTY-EIGHT—SUNDAY

For becoming more aware of HOW TO KEEP MYSELF FROM SMOKING—

Today I will work on my *Higher Thinking Center* with material from the following dreams:

We are now completing four weeks of work on our goal of HOW TO KEEP OURSELF FROM SMOKING. We are hopefully going from some point of reaction-ambivalence to limited willingness. Perhaps we are willing to do whatever it takes, but not a smidgen more. Perhaps it is with this limited willingness that we have a dream like the following:

> There is an incident where we get an order for a small steel plate from a potential customer and are going to try and run it out and there is some question from

> one of the girls working about whether we should also give him a little gift. We say, 'No.' That would embarrass him. He would be overwhelmed with not only the service but the gift and have a sort of reverse reaction. Better to just give him the plate.

Perhaps that is true. All we really want is the 'plate.' On the other hand, we may need to deal with things relating to our particular center and our particular habit. Part of our 'cure' might deal with recognition of these things. As an example, perhaps we also have the following dream on this night or early morning:

> We are at the office early and see a responsible employee come in fifteen minutes late. We seem a bit uncomfortable being there at that time, but for some reason, are. We say something to someone after an incident—'There's one thing this place doesn't have is a shortage of tempers!'

Also during this night or early morning we have a couple of quick dream statements that go as follows:

> 'Every top will be accounted for.'

> Power Over To New. (A headline)

Does 'Every top will be accounted for' mean that every time we blow our top we will account for it? Perhaps it also might mean that every success (as KEEPING OURSELF FROM SMOKING) is accounted for (whereas we can forget every failure, and 'slips' do not count). By spending a day or so working on this kind of sentence, saying it repeatedly, the meanings it might have would amaze us.

'Power Over To New': Does this concede our willingness to give our energy over to the new idea of KEEPING OURSELF FROM SMOKING? Part of the pleasure and challenge in this work is finding the answer for ourself. We can share with others, if we dare, but there can be very little that equals a meaningful phrase that becomes part of our innermost life.

We may be completing another spiraling upward ascent toward our goal. Even if we still have some misgivings, we may refute it as quickly as in the following dream:

> Some image where a wife says something to her husband about it won't work—she is standing at the door and he is on the sidewalk. It almost seems as if someone else might show up when she shuts the door.

DAY TWENTY-NINE—MONDAY

For becoming more aware of HOW TO KEEP MYSELF FROM SMOKING—

Today I will work on my *Instinctive Center* with material from the following dreams:

What we never really seem to understand, though we would probably all suspect it if we took a moment to consider, are the little ways we protest decisions forced upon us. We may protest by our subtleness or not so subtle actions, our behavior, and we may protest by what we feel or what we think. When we work with our dreams as we try to improve some aspect of ourself— here, becoming more aware of HOW TO KEEP OURSELF FROM SMOKING—we have to be patient with all the shenanigans we are liable to pull. We just have to look upon ourself as a rebellious hoodlum or tyke. It is not that we are evil. We are just human. So, what we might see is this sort of dream:

> There is a dream where we make some kind of deal to roll a couple of cigarettes for someone for a price or have someone else roll them. We set up the time and the place and then we are not sure if we have the paper and the tobacco. But the other guy seems to have it all. Then the guy appears and the other fellow is going to do it, though it looks like perhaps someone else has come earlier.

It might almost sound to some of us as if we are listening to some adventure of Tom Sawyer. Further, another dream seems to admit a kind of helplessness on our part:

> There is a dream where we seem to have some guy out to see someone who seems to owe money, we think. We also have a policeman out too. We also look at a building outside that has some funny words on it. Like 'Nekud' or something. We remember telling the policeman we can not help, but he can.

By patiently allowing for all of this material to play itself out, we are earning the right to be free of it. If we protest the actual playing of the material, then we forfeit the right to be free. We may look free and manage to act free, but we will not be free. Perhaps, we even have a one sentence dream that goes as follows:

With a gloomy bunch as you are . . .

Yes, that may be because we are not feeling great. We have risked much time and still we may not have anything tangible. Feeling really happy is hard, but it is all a process. When we see a play, read a book, watch a movie, we are taken through all sorts of 'transitions,' and when we work on our dreams, we experience our own transitions.

We are also getting the benefit of some kind of reward for our effort. Perhaps we can even take that 'gloomy bunch' line and convert it into some syncopated beat that will convert our gloominess into hopefulness and good cheer. Tapping a foot or clapping hands can help us even further.

DAY THIRTY—TUESDAY

For becoming more aware of HOW TO KEEP MYSELF FROM SMOKING—

Today I will work on my *Sexual Center* with material from the following dreams:

Have we been working on our dreams with the tools we discussed a few days ago? Are we trying to focus on our goal of becoming more aware of HOW TO KEEP OURSELF FROM SMOKING, as we go to sleep? Are we also keeping in mind the particular center that we are working on, as we go to sleep? Repeating the little statement THREE TIMES each time we think of it may be worthwhile. Repeat it as we lie down to sleep, and even as we awaken during the night and early morning. Repetition allows our mind to know that we mean business. We are sincere about what we are doing, and we want to impress whatever needs impressing that we are after a certain kind of knowledge.

Further, are we trying to remember the two separate ideas, the idea of becoming aware of HOW TO KEEP OURSELF FROM SMOKING and the idea of the particular center, as we review our dreams and try to get some sort of experience from them?

If we make the efforts mentioned above, perhaps we have a dream like the following, or at least something that lets us know that we are on the right track :

> There's a dream where we seem to go to the top of some theater and stand up on the structure and eat something and sort of grab hard on the structure with our knees to keep from falling. Once it looks like we might, but we hang on. We think we are eating raisins. Before, we hear a couple of young undergraduates talking and kidding each other about their works being reviewed and if they have bought the reviews.

We are now able to begin getting something quite specific. We are advancing in a way that several weeks ago might have seemed unthinkable. We are getting images in our mind that give us strength to continue our quest. Also we are now more open, hopefully to a full blast of reality concerning our smoking, that perhaps we could not have handled before.

We may then have a dream that clearly lays it on the line about how we are somehow missing the reality of what we are engaged in. Since this may occur in the *Sexual Center* we might need to be prepared for something so ridiculous that we cannot help but begin replacing the images of smoking that we have carried around with us for so long—images of happy people conversing and celebrating in interesting places, glimpses of attractive people doing hearty and courageous acts in ways that arouse a certain respect or admiration from us. These new images project a total absence on our part of reality, conscience and productivity. Such may then be the following sort of dream we have. We share it because of the effect it has on us, not because of its contents:

> We're witnessing an act of 'intercourse' between two men who have no business being together. One is on top and he seems to have a vagina. The door is closed to the room and they are 'doing it.' Every so often the one on top says, "That's enough," but the one on the bottom insists they go on since he is about ready to come. But he's gotten soft—then slowly hard, but in the end he doesn't climax. All the time they are doing it, the one on the bottom does not seem to think anything is wrong or odd.

The problem with this sort of dream is that we can override it with our reason, censor it, and promptly forget it. Then we are the loser. It is not something to experience once and lay aside. It is a doctrine of disclosure. It needs restatement with the goal we have chosen and the particular center with which we are working. We need to respect its shock value as a way of impressing upon us something that we need to know. Just as we need this sort of shock, we also need finer disclosures that hopefully now will begin to appear.

DAY THIRTY-ONE—WEDNESDAY

For becoming more aware of HOW TO KEEP MYSELF FROM SMOKING—

Today I will work on my *Moving Center* with material from the following dreams:

We may expect certain things from our dreams, once we reach what we think is a new understanding, let us say, of the severity of our smoking habit. We may look forward to new information and get something that we have not anticipated. Dreams operate differently than we might imagine. Logic and rational expectation do not always figure prominently in dreams. However, we should never turn away from them, as if they are a waste of time. Part of the value of dreams is that they force us to look at something in a way that we might not want to, but need to.

In the following dream, we might be experiencing a distancing of ourself from something that we were a part of before.

> We are going up an alley at night—fairly late—and we hear some sounds coming from a meeting of people we were once close to. Now we seem to feel almost distant from what they are doing.

Isn't this, perhaps, a similar feeling to how we may feel abandoning our 'friends'—the 'cigarettes' or 'cigars?' We may also notice the very strong contrast between 'going up a dark alley' and not being 'inside with all the so-called cheer.' Isn't that also how we might be feeling now, as we go up this alley (not really knowing how it will end)? Some danger is involved, although standing still is dangerous also.

Perhaps, we have another dream on this night or early morning, which again is different from what we might have been expecting:

> We seem to be out of a meeting and an old acquaintance draws our attention to money and some kind of sandwiches on a table and says, "Don't eat anything that has blood in or on it." It seems like a warning about disease. We then each seem to get a packet of money. We leave ours on a chair in a folder while we go out for a moment. Then we worry about someone perhaps taking some of the bills. We think there are fifty—but suppose there aren't or some disappear? We also take a big sandwich or cake. Then we are outside trying to get across the street and sort of directing someone who happens to be crossing. We hear someone singing something and sort of comment out loud toward him.

Perhaps we may not know how to deal with this sort of dream. Particularly the admonition about 'Don't eat anything that has blood in or on it.' We may turn away from this sort of thing. After all, all we are after is a way to KEEP OURSELF FROM SMOKING. It may be that such an admonition might never appear in a dream. If such a thing does appear, however, it probably behooves us at least to hold it up for consideration. There may be a correlation between diet and not smoking which would help us considerably.

Ultimately, we have to simply accept the unexpectedness that is part of dreams and be willing to record them however odd or unwanted they may be. The very thing that we scoff at initially, we may learn to be very grateful for later.

DAY THIRTY-TWO—THURSDAY

For becoming more aware of HOW TO KEEP MYSELF FROM SMOKING—

Today I will work on my *Emotional Center* with material from the following dreams:

One nice thing about dreaming only one dream, and a short one at that, is that we have all the time we might be allotting to this project to spend on just the one dream. Often this gives us sufficient time really to work with it. The following is the only dream that we have last night:

> There is something about finding some broken glass in the sink that we have not noticed before—broken by someone other than us this time. We begin to realize that we are breaking a lot of glass lately. Also we notice that the trash container has invoices under it as well as a bunch of oranges. There is actually a hole in the container.

Now, as we work with this dream, we can not help but feel that a person who breaks much glass is a klutz. We do not think of ourselves as a klutz, but there is no point in arguing with a dream. What we do not think we are is often precisely what we are.

Of course, someone else may have a very different sense and experience with this dream. The only thing that matters is what we as individuals sense. That is the only thing that makes the whole thing worthwhile. If we try to fudge, we lose the punch of it.

Yet just to leave it at that, that we are a klutz, does not really do much. We are trying to become as aware as we can of HOW TO KEEP OURSELF FROM SMOKING, and we need to try to align our dreams with the focus we are trying to maintain. So what kind of klutz are we? Could it be that we are suddenly realizing that emotionally, as a smoker, we are a klutz? The image of broken glass in the sink then becomes an image of how we really treat ourself when we smoke: very stupidly. Can we connect that way? Sometimes we have to draw ourself closer and closer to the point, almost as if we are pulling a stubborn mule to a trough. It is one foot at a time, slowly and patiently. Then when we finally get it to the trough, we gently nudge its face toward the water. Perhaps, we need to say quietly, 'We love you, although you are such a klutz!'

There is more to the dream, and with time we can work with it. The image of invoices underneath a trash container may not reek of klutzdom, but it surely strikes us as the height of carelessness. After all, invoices are the juice of a business. If we do not send them to customers, how long can a business last? To see them deposited beneath a trash container seems terribly self-immolating. Again, criticism of our work competence needs to have a particular focus and, here again we are working with KEEPING OURSELF FROM SMOKING. So we have another image of how we treat ourself emotionally when we smoke—it is like throwing away invoices.

The image of a bunch of oranges, which we may particularly cherish as a daily supplement to our diet, underneath the same trash container, simply tells us again that as a smoker, emotionally we are throwing away some of the best nourishment we have. Finally, we may take some solace from the idea that there is a hole in the bottom, which perhaps shows that both the invoices and the oranges are not totally lost. By our effort, at least, they are close to being rediscovered and picked up.

Once we finish with this sort of work, let us sit back for a moment and just go over the dream again, not with our head, but with our heart and back. Let us try to make all of this effort a part of our new thinking process. We are working with such incredibly sophisticated tools, when we work with our mind and heart and moving center, we can feel confident that with our new ideas, a very different result will emerge than 'smoking as usual.'

DAY THIRTY-THREE—FRIDAY

For becoming more aware of HOW TO KEEP MYSELF FROM SMOKING—

Today I will work on my *Thinking Center* with material from the following dreams:

When we go to sleep immediately upon going to bed, without even having a moment to say, "For becoming more aware of/HOW TO KEEP MYSELF FROM SMOKING/Tomorrow I will work on my *Think-*

ing Center/with material from the following dreams"—when we are asleep even before we have said this—then when we do awaken with a dream, often it is a bit jumbled. This is not as clear a remembering as we normally have. In such a case, we get the flavor or sense of the dream, but can hardly reconstruct it.

Such a dream is the following, where we are talking with some old classmates and they are saying what they are going to be doing this coming weekend. We get the feeling that there is something particularly appealing in their invitation to join them. Nothing is really said outright, but when we awaken and feel so good about what has occurred, it begins to dawn on us that all these classmates no longer smoke. Their invitation to us is really one of joining the life style they now enjoy.

It is probably very difficult to convey the 'new feeling' we have with this sort of dream. It goes over and beyond the content and seems to transport us to a new kind of feeling about the way we live. On the other hand, having awakened and reminded ourself of the commitment we have about becoming more aware of HOW TO KEEP OURSELF FROM SMOKING, we might have a very different sort of dream:

> There is a dream where two men are waiting for Hitler to appear. We see men outside and then we see a parade of several vehicles followed by a huge limousine ten times larger than any we have seen and we see its driver and then, far at the rear we glimpse a figure and it seems some words like 'savior,' 'guide.' The men meanwhile seem to be getting ready to meet this person.

There might be much fear exhibited by one of the two men, as he turns to the other and he seems impressed that this second man knows Hitler. But the extremely ridiculous length of the limousine, so far out of normal human proportion to the driver and passenger, gives it a sense of sheer absurdity. And the words 'savior,' 'guide' seem more imagined than palpable.

Having a dream about Hitler is one thing, but recognizing that we cannot just scoff at this villain and be done with it is another. Dreams often reveal two truths. One is the obvious one of poking fun at the so-called person paraded. Still, the other is to let us know that there must be something about us that is like Hitler. The second aspect, we do not particularly like dealing with but, of course, that is the whole point. So what do we have here? We are working with the idea of becoming more aware of HOW TO KEEP OURSELF FROM SMOKING, and we are dealing with the *Thinking Center.* When we think of Hitler, we think of his angry speeches, his voice in a frenzy and how he got people to think of him as a savior, a guide.

Is there some part of ourself that is like that? In German, 'Mein Fuhrer' (My Leader) sounds pretty close to 'my furor' in English, and we have to admit that there is in our thinking a tendency to furor. Do we tend to let this 'furor' be our savior, our guide, when it comes to forcing us to grab for a cigarette? Do we not let this furor go unabated—almost allow it to control our life in part?

We are not particularly proud of this furor of ours, but there might be an aspect of awe with which the rest of us regards it. Perhaps our smoking became somehow wrapped up with it as we went from adolescence to adulthood. There was a 'strength' about the furor, and we always thought there was a similar 'masculine strength' in puffing on a cigarette. Now it seems like Hitler—absurd and very dangerous.

The last dream we have on this night or early morning goes as follows:

Also some headlines:
US OIL PROPERTIES DISCOVERED

When we work on our awareness of HOW TO KEEP OURSELF FROM SMOKING and we work on our *Thinking Center*, we are doing the equivalent of discovering oil properties.

We may ask: How much longer? How much do we have to work before we can KEEP OURSELF FROM SMOKING?

Many of us have been smoking for a lifetime, or at least for many years. We are trying to come up with a harmonious awareness that will deal with all those years of smoking. Many of us need to iterate the ideas that are expressed and experienced, perhaps differently, by our different centers. We need to rebuild our thinking and feeling and all the other things that impinge on our smoking. If it takes another two weeks, can we wait?

DAY THIRTY-FOUR—SATURDAY

For becoming more aware of HOW TO KEEP MYSELF FROM SMOKING—

Today I will work on my *Higher Emotional Center* with material from the following dreams:

How are we doing with our dreams? Are we getting some results? We need to apply ourself as much as we can and rest assured that we will achieve something for our efforts. For some of us, it may be just one thing that sets us in motion to KEEP OURSELF FROM

SMOKING. For others, it may be the kind of thing that we are enduring together as we record every night. For some it will be a combination. There is no way of predicting who will take one way, who will take another, but we do believe that guidance will be provided with the method we are describing.

As we said initially, or at least implied, working with dreams is working with a new language and working with new experiences. We have to take risks as we go—with sensing what is being said.

As we have probably found out by now, some dreams are figurative, some are literal and some a combination of the two. Following is a figurative one that we dream on this night or early morning:

> There is a dream where we see a casket being removed from a movie theater.

We have a hard time with this dream. There is not a lot to 'sense,' and we really are not sure what to make of it. Yet, as we try to work with this dream, both keeping in mind the idea of the *Higher Emotional Center* and HOW TO KEEP OURSELF FROM SMOKING—we find ourself risking the thought that what we are seeing is 'death' in the midst of 'entertainment,' and perhaps that is precisely what we risk when we smoke.

Still, what we find is that after having said that, we still need to go back to the image and repeat often the 'seeing' of the casket being removed from a movie theater. For, ultimately, it is our emotional sense of what we are doing that is going to have a big part in KEEPING US FROM SMOKING.

On the other hand, what can we say about the following two 'literal' dreams that we have?

> It seems we are sitting at a table and a woman appears and says something about sticking our hand in our mouth to avert fatigue—though she does not just say it plainly but sort of infers it.
>
> We seem to be talking to an old friend and his wife and we say, 'When someone ruffles our feelings we should say, 'F--k you' (inside) and not let it bother us.'

"Yuck," may be our response and perhaps rightly so. Yet we are trying to work on the idea of becoming more aware of HOW TO KEEP OURSELF FROM SMOKING, and if we happen to smoke partly when fatigue and partly when our feelings are ruffled, perhaps there is some wisdom here for us alone. Next to our thoughts, dreams are the most private affairs we indulge in, so we can use them however we so elect. Perhaps after the first and second rejection, we might turn to such dreams and find some solace, some guidance.

Such dreams may not be the 'finished products' of our being, but only the 'work in process' information that will gradually make us into something noteworthy. If we have to be a bit shocked or upset during this 'work in process' stage, to move our life along in a noteworthy way, what of it? Would we not (as individuals), in the privacy of our own life, prefer to deal with the ugliness and distastefulness of our smoking NOW, in order to be free and more wholesome LATER? Is there really one of us who is so 'turned off' by a temporary coarseness in our dreams that we would rather continue unchanged?

Given the smallest taste of new knowledge, the tiniest hint of a better way, have we a choice other than to hang in there? We owe it not only to ourself but also to our service as a human being.

DAY THIRTY-FIVE—SUNDAY

For becoming more aware of HOW TO KEEP MYSELF FROM SMOKING—

Today I will work on my *Higher Thinking Center* with material from the following dreams:

There is no gainsaying our dreams. We simply cannot be, much as we probably would like to be, masters over them. We *can* set up a process where we feed certain thoughts to whatever starts them and by that receive some pertinent information. But often it is not what we 'want,' frequently it is not what we 'like,' but always (we believe) it is what we 'need.' That is why we affirm our constancy in the present process we are engaged in: Becoming more aware of HOW TO KEEP OURSELF FROM SMOKING, by working with our particular centers with material we dream.

Nevertheless, we have been at it for THIRTY-FIVE DAYS. We have targeted our journey's end in another two weeks. So with hope and a little trepidation, we may ask: What is next? Dreams do not necessarily answer in the same key that we ask. But they do answer.

Let us see what last night's or this early morning's dreams might say:

> There is some sort of workout at the office by an esoteric movement group and the visiting instructor from out of town is apparently going back. He sits at the table and notices some sort of model we have made and we seem to discuss something with him. We then ask him or

> allude to what he will do next—and he doesn't seem to say. He seems very thin in the arms. We seem to want to refer to that thing we have just found in our dream journal about when people appear in dreams: (Some girl is talking to a guy and saying that he represents a certain something to her and when in her mind she is struggling with something he seems to help her just by her thinking of him. It seems to remind us of how dreams will suddenly show someone and we wonder why they are there. Perhaps at that particular time and moment we need them there.)

So what we think we want—information on what the instructor will do next—we do not get; yet what we do not think we want—but apparently need—is some information on how we should regard people who are in our dreams. Perhaps there is something 'comforting' in knowing that people appear in our dreams BECAUSE WE NEED THEM THERE.

Another quick dream we have goes as follows:

> Some sign posts on the roof top instead of smoke stacks.

Perhaps we HAVE eliminated smoking and are now in pursuit of MEANINGFUL GUIDANCE.

But, again, we do not seem to get what we want:

> . . . We seem to be wandering around, first we get to a point like a bridge-approaching city street where we are afraid

> to go down some sort of unspecific steps, and find another way, but then we are in pajamas and go back. Then we start again and think we see an old classmate but it is some look-alike who seems to sniff at us and ask if we have worked in the Far East. Then another guy asks, "Got any ideas?" We laugh—"About what?" "Well"—he begins and launches into some sort of tirade about something. We leave him and ask where the place is where we have been before—and someone says The Omar and we start out again.

So on and on we go and perhaps we should relax and know that we are safe. Perhaps some of us are not experiencing this sort of thing. Others are doing just fine. We would like to think that whatever our individual situation, all of us remain determined to keep on, gathering information. Some of it may seem beside the point, but all of it we apparently need, as we continue.

DAY THIRTY-SIX—MONDAY

For becoming more aware of HOW TO KEEP MYSELF FROM SMOKING—

Today I will work on my *Instinctive Center* with material from the following dreams:

> We seem to be in England and some guy's head is in a bag on top of the ground and he sees us and with glaring eyes, says: "Why don't you do something?"—and we say: 'Suppose we kick

your head off?" It is cheeky but he is cheeky—and we are impatient. We also talk about how in England, they make some kind of bomb that can blow off a guy's feet and they don't seem to get too upset.

Will we be able to recognize in this dream a particularly negative strain, which may have come from the persistent struggle we have been making to become aware of HOW TO KEEP OURSELF FROM SMOKING? We have an edge to our disposition, which seems to make us appear as if we do not care what happens. We do, of course. But what we do see more clearly than before is how much we seem to be lacking in love. And it is in this reflection that we find ourself wanting to adjust the manner in which we are going on this journey. Somehow, in the pursuit of finding a way to KEEP OURSELF FROM SMOKING, we have overlooked a special factor that has appeared in various dreams over the years.

That factor is love. Love often gets left out of our formulas in life, yet it just might be that love IS the formula. And over the years the following four admonishments to love have appeared in our dreams:

Love is the universal elixir.

Fill your mind and heart with love.

If we can look at someone
and love them, and not be so
concerned with inner thinking
about (my name) . . . myself . . .
myself . . . (my name) . . .

We have to love things
as we also find ourself
reacting against them.

So what we now propose is to amend our nightly pre-slumber statement to read as follows (and starting with this Monday night): 'For becoming more and more aware/(through love)/ of HOW TO KEEP MYSELF FROM SMOKING / tomorrow I will work on my *Sexual Center* / with material from the following dreams:'

If we could remember to include the four admonishments to love on the heels of our nightly statement—perhaps that would also help. Of course, who can merely *say* something and expect immediate results? But if we try, we will find that part of ourself which responds most readily to our persistent need and always shows mercy when mercy is due.

DAY THIRTY-SEVEN—TUESDAY

For becoming more and more aware (through love) of HOW TO KEEP MYSELF FROM SMOKING—

Today I will work on my *Sexual Center* with material from the following dreams:

Are we spending time on our dreams, somehow? Life can be brutally hard on our time choices and personal disciplines, but we always need to be looking for an opening. Perhaps when we least expect it, there will be time during the day for us to snatch a few moments to spend on our dreams. For it does take a little time. The experiences we have in dreams often do not mean much until we have reviewed them for a while.

On the other hand, occasionally a dream is obvious and perhaps a mite witty. Maybe wittier than we might like. Perhaps we have such a dream as the following in the night or early morning:

> There's a dream where someone is asking us about the steel business as far as getting things to the job—and we say if we can get the steel joists, metal deck and fabricated structural steel all on the job at the same time, then the erection is no big deal. It goes fine.

If we put aside any impulse to laugh at a fear in this particular center and focus on how we might understand this dream in the light of wanting to become aware of HOW TO KEEP OURSELF FROM SMOKING, we can perhaps draw some strength from the idea expressed that the actual act of NOT SMOKING is no big deal. It is the idea that we need to assemble all the necessary components before we can expect to be successful. We need to have some kind of willingness and strength, which hopefully we are getting through the work that we are currently doing. Next, we need to find the right time and maybe even the right place. Perhaps we can find out more about these last two items later. Nevertheless, we do not want to BEGIN TO KEEP OURSELF FROM SMOKING, when we are under tremendous stress and in a place where such a beginning would be doomed from its inception.

Perhaps a symbolic key or two might help us if we dream something like the following:

> There is also a dream where we go to pick up a couple who are old friends of ours. They have moved from their house to a smaller house. When we open the door we see the husband sitting, almost meditating, and the living room is not all straightened up and startling, sort of plain. Then we start to go someplace and we are not sure what the husband is talking about when he refers to something—and we are not sure if the way we're going is the way he wants to go.

Again, we are experiencing, perhaps, our own 'unknowingness' by experiencing the 'unknowingness' of the dream. At least, we become conscious of this 'unknowingness' and have to struggle with it, as opposed to not even knowing THAT we do not know.

The next dream that we have in this center goes as follows:

> Something about #1 being health and happiness.

This is the sort of 'wisdom' that we might want to put on our 'personal wisdom card.' It is not that it is something that no one has ever uttered before, but it might just be something that WE have never said to ourself before. As such, it is wisdom that now BELONGS to us.

It is such a simple statement that we believe it can help us immeasurably in getting to the root of what we really want out of life. IF we in fact do dream such a statement, then we might seriously want to see if we are currently living accordingly. If we are still a smoker, we might want to examine that first word (health) and see if in fact there can be smoking and health concurrently in our life.

If we find that such cannot be—that there is no way to have health and be a smoker—then we have further ammunition in which we can discharge our individual responsibility to ourself and our family. After all, WHO was it that got us to smoke? Weren't we small or immature when it really happened? Did we really exercise any choice at the time? Who are we now? If we now see that #1 is health and happiness, we now see what we need to do.

We should, however, be cautious about pressuring ourself. To know what we should do is one thing and to know when and how is another. We will learn when and how in due time, if we continue.

DAY THIRTY-EIGHT—WEDNESDAY

For becoming more and more aware (through love) of HOW TO KEEP MYSELF FROM SMOKING—

Today I will work on my *Moving Center* with material from the following dreams:

Imagine, we have been together for THIRTY-EIGHT DAYS, working on an idea that has little common sense, but tremendous inner power. It is as if we decided to set sail for a part of the world we have never visited, nor ever really spoken of with anyone else who has either. We have few maps and very primitive conveyances. They give us very little direction and we really must operate on faith and hope.

Yet, perhaps we are finding some moments that are very different from our usual living moments. Perhaps we are getting, occasionally, some clue as to what might be within us that could help KEEP OURSELF FROM SMOKING.

We would be the first to admit that this whole thing could be a marvelously funny skit. We could have great fun with it ourself. Still, the fact that we are so vulnerable to comedy does not really take away from the fact that the work we are doing can be very important for us.

Of course, there IS something funny in sophisticated men and women of the early twenty-first century resorting to something so basic as an examination of their dreams. Haven't we got beyond that sort of thing? Apparently, we have in many respects, but there is a void that 'other people's knowledge' has for us; it just cannot quite give us what we need when it comes to solving some personal problems. We are forced to become, again, primitive man, wrestling with his dreams, only now working with them according to some sort of formula.

So how are we doing with this formula? Are we able to look at our dreams, after careful thought, and try with as much energy as we have, to inculcate our mind with what is being said? Do we have any sort of result trying to line up our desire to KEEP OURSELF FROM SMOKING, and the particular center we are dreaming in? Does ANYTHING fall into place?

'Meaning' just might be that thought or feeling or sense of truth that suddenly occurs 'between' these two poles of study. Let us examine what is a dream for us—like the following:

> Something about being at a big castle and seeing some sort of baronial table cloth and finding ourself inscribing something on it with one of the words being 'ambrosial' and then the man at the head

> of it cautions us, without knowing we have already written on it, against writing anything on it. Shortly after, we ask him if we can have one of the cloths, that was very pretty, and had some sort of designs on it, and he agrees a bit hesitantly. Someone else seems to think he may want some information on it. Then the head man of the place, perhaps a duke or something, appears and we, having heard he is a chef, ask him if he is and he says "No"—but he has apparently had some chef's courses. He is a sailor-like fellow and is scooping up and away several large desserts that have not yet been consumed. One is a huge raw peanut thing—and he seems to be destroying it and putting it all in a bowl.

How diligently are we able to work with this sort of dream? It is a very different place from where we are used to being. This richness probably is not duplicatable. Yet something comes through, that lives, that is trying to show us how to live. Nevertheless, it just hints at it, doesn't it? Yet if we can try to keep alive the images that we receive in this sort of dream, perhaps 'new paths are made in our current brain,' and something will draw on us eventually. We may not even 'link it' to this dream; we might just suddenly understand what we are supposed to do. Part of the dream might be telling us something about food, and how we handle it now, and what we should begin instructing ourself to do with it. Food is the subject in this next dream also:

> Being somewhere and saying that frozen brussel sprouts seem better than the others if they are not cooked so long. Also someone seems to be eating corn on a plate with lettuce. We see the remnants of a birthday cake and start to eat a piece but would like to stop remembering 'we are what we eat.'

We are what we eat. Have you heard that before? Perhaps, but we may not have thought that it needed to be heeded too strongly. We may have said, "Yes . . . but maybe no . . ." Now we are perhaps forced to make it a part of our own understanding.

Often, we are very lax about these ideas. We cannot just believe that they would really make any difference in our life. Still, it is precisely these sorts of ideas that are the ONLY WAY there can be a difference in our life. Paying attention to these 'tips' is the beginning of being able to change.

We need to be able to allow ourself a little living space to experiment with these new ideas. We need to be willing to take a small risk, initially, and try some things mentioned in our dreams. Maybe KEEPING OURSELF FROM SMOKING begins with 'trying some new ideas,' WITHOUT even STOPPING at first. Maybe, something begins to happen to us inwardly, and the faint idea of KEEPING OURSELF FROM SMOKING, thanks to our trying a few things, really takes hold and happens.

Each of us will know how it works when we give it a chance TO work.

DAY THIRTY-NINE—THURSDAY

For becoming more and more aware (through love) of HOW TO KEEP MYSELF FROM SMOKING—

Today I will work on my *Emotional Center* with material from the following dreams:

We may find as we go on this journey, that for some reason or other, we are less troubled with some centers' dreams than with others'; or we are more interested in some centers' dreams than in others. One center which may trouble us more than the others is the Emotional Center.

If we have a hard time with 'emotions', we may find that this is one center that we almost want to get PAST. The following example shows us that the Emotional Center might be less developed and therefore in need of niore time and attention than any of the other centers:

> There is some meeting at someone's house and it seems a childhood friend is involved. Also, we think an employee of ours may want an extra ten days for something.

That extra ten days could well be referring to the time between now and the end of our journey. Hopefully by then, we should have the tools to enable us to start KEEPING OURSELF FROM SMOKING. But for now, we concede a kind of slowness which forces us to admit that we are not going to be emotionally resolute until the end of the fifty days allotted to us.

Again, the next dream points to a difficulty we may be having:

> 'Once we know their credit, we are going to do it.' The scene is some customer talking about what he is going to do, and we seem to be a little hesitant, but our superintendent says the right thing.

Often dreams speak on several levels of truth. In a business sense, knowing someone's credit allows us to do business with them. Nevertheless, what is really being spoken of here is our own credit. It is realizing that once we know OUR OWN CREDIT, we can probably do IT. We probably do not feel too confident about our own credit, if we dream this sort of dream. Our 'superintendent' seems to know but the rest of us—or at least the part in question, our *Emotional Center*—is 'hesitant.'

How can we change, become more confident? Recognizing that we *are not* confident right now, might be a start. By repeating this little phrase and trying to keep in mind our particular center, the *Emotional Center*, and our goal, HOW TO KEEP OURSELF FROM SMOKING, we might drill a new attitude into ourself.

Just to say the phrase—'Once we know their credit, we are going to do it'—without trying to bring in the *Emotional Center* and our Goal, is not infusing it with specificity. Yet to say it with those two things in mind may not only infuse the phrase but really give us some inner nourishment.

Some of us may have another dream—similar to the one that follows:

> We are in some place and a guy is putting his hands on us, and we say: 'Get your f--king hands off!'—instead of being understanding. He may even be a bit retarded.

We need to love things as we also find ourself reacting against them. There is no better way to begin than by trying to inculcate this in a dream. If we cannot do it when we dream, at least do it, or try to do it, after the dream, when we are reflecting on it. We need to recognize that love is not some luxury that people may or may not have at their discretion. It is an absolute necessity and something we have to cultivate if we are going to be successful with our dreams.

When we cool off from our inflammatory remarks to the 'bit retarded' guy, we might realize that perhaps we are such, ourself. Not that we really BELIEVE IT, but at least we can try again to visualize the scene, try to recall the guy's hands putting themselves on us, and hear ourself getting terribly offended as we say what we said. Then try to see that perhaps our rejection of him is really our rejection of our own humanity as well.

These things are exercises that we can do, in the privacy of our own mind and heart, without hurting any living soul or disturbing any of our present life style. What we will receive for our efforts will be a 'better' harmony of all of our centers—particularly the ones that we are weak in—and a realization of our goal of knowing HOW TO KEEP OURSELF FROM SMOKING.

DAY FORTY—FRIDAY

For becoming more and more aware (through love) of HOW TO KEEP MYSELF FROM SMOKING—

Today I will work on my *Thinking Center* with material from the following dreams:

Another center that may be giving us a little trouble is the *Thinking Center*. Here again, we may be finding a certain 'something' that tells us that we are not really confident about achieving our goal.

Perhaps we have a dream similar to the following:

> Some attractive blond living in an apartment building we are apparently living in asks us if she can borrow fifty dollars. We say, 'Yes.' Then she says, "How about one hundred dollars or two fifty dollars?" We say, 'No.' Then we go back to get the money and see an old friend who has just returned real ragged looking from a trip, and we ask him if we should get her driver's license. "No, not this time." 'Not this time?' we say, inferring suppose she runs out on us? But he tries to say that women have not had a franchise for borrowing. They apparently deserve a chance.

This is perhaps our own predicament, if we have dreamed a dream similar to this one. We doubt our own credit worthiness. We are afraid to extend credit to ourself. Perhaps it is strange for us to realize that a part of us is reluctant to be confident about something we are trying to do, while other parts may be quite sympathetic and willing. This is precisely why we have such a hard time with ourself, seeing with one part of ourself the necessity of doing something, while another part or parts may not seem to want to extend to us the 'credit energy' to go full steam ahead.

Once we begin to see this phenomenon, we begin to work with ourself with as much patience as we can muster. HOW TO KEEP OURSELF FROM SMOKING begins to look like a problem that requires more than coercion or fear or even consternation. We are up against a condition of being human that calls for as much 'dexterity in our thinking and focusing' as we can promulgate among our various parts.

We may even have a further put-down as we lay half way between sleep and awakening. We may mini-dream the following:

> Anything you say is hard to believe.

What do we do with this sort of negativity? We need to first recognize that it is true, in some respect. It is an honest expression from this part of ourself and, as such, it needs to be taken seriously. It reflects a long established lack of 'credibility' in this part of ourself in relationship to our other parts. Perhaps sometime long ago (who knows . . . who really cares . . .) there was some sort of betrayal, something that just hurt and created this negative situation. On the other hand, 'hard to believe' does not mean 'isn't possible' or 'will not work.' It just means what it says, 'It is hard.'

Perhaps some sort of 'conversation' with our *Thinking Center* would help, or at least get us to begin dealing with this very 'honest' yet 'difficult' center.

> '*Thinking Center*, we want you to know that we desperately need to have your support and honesty as we try to become aware of how to keep ourself from smoking. We are sorry for anything that

> might have occurred in the past. Perhaps we put you through the ringer on a few occasions, when we were young and more impetuous than we are even now. You've been hurt by some other part of us. We are sorry. We need your help. We are going to try to undo something that has been a real curse for us. We are going to KEEP OURSELF FROM SMOKING. We know that you can help. You know us as well as any part, and you have the honesty, we have noticed, to cut through a lot of 'vague and unsuitable ideas' that may come to us in weak moments or from others (who are different from us). So please give us a chance; give us the credit to work on this idea and help us in any way you can.'

Possibly, after such a plea, we may find or imagine our *Thinking Center* saying:

> "I will do what I can. Certainly, your goal is admirable and your current situation is deplorable. Listen to what I say and do not try to overlook your general improvement—because you cannot do this thing, just by itself."

DAY FORTY-ONE—SATURDAY

For becoming more and more aware (through love) of HOW TO KEEP MYSELF FROM SMOKING—

Today I will work on my *Higher Emotional Center* with material from the following dreams:

Dreams have a way of bringing up subjects that often get overlooked by our so-called conscious mind. Often what they say tends to put things in a perspective which not only helps us considerably but also can avoid misunderstandings later. This is perhaps the value of the following dream that we experience during the night or early morning:

> We seem to be at some special group outing and some guy comes along and wants to see if we can make him some mashed potatoes and corn bread. We say, 'Yes,' thinking we can just do it ourself with a recipe we have. Then he says, 'What about grits?' We say, 'Yes'—thinking we can do that for him too, and charge about $5.95. But then we ask a girl to do it—since we realize we don't have the recipes with us. She says she is busy. Then we asked the group leader and she says, 'No, it can ruin us.' Then she starts to explain how someone made something for someone before and it practically ruined the group. Then it dawns on us, we can be liable for anything we fix—and we see the wisdom in not fixing anything.

We want everyone to realize at this stage of the game that everything written here is only for others' proper use. It in no way makes the claim for anything other than a possible guide for becoming aware of HOW TO KEEP FROM SMOKING.

Still, it is not a recipe for 'definite success.' We should view it as one views a physical exercise program. If one has 'problems of some sort,' then perhaps consultation with one's 'problem helper' would be in order. If one is eager to adapt the words here for other pursuits, we cannot say anything either way.

We feel that we have all been given the gift of dreams and it should be accepted with a certain deference. We should NOT TRY TO DO ANYTHING, without careful consideration. If we happen to dream of climbing a very steep mountain, we should not rent mountaineering gear and start out, without some careful reflection: Have we ever climbed a mountain before? Are we not going off half-cocked before we really understand what is being said? Care needs to be taken with all such things. We need to exercise judgment and retain some sense of humor. A dream that identifies us as a 'zilch' by some member of our family may be a very true description of us, but we should not take out after the particular member of the family with some vengeful spirit. He or she could be absolutely innocent. If they do 'think' what we dream, so what? We are after truth in any guise we may find it, and 'not out to set things straight.'

So let us continue our journey with a better understanding of what we are about. Many new ideas may be given to us and some may surprise us greatly. Whether we should take them literally or merely reflect on them as some sort of 'inner aspect of ourself'—we have to decide.

Perhaps, at a later stage in our life, we catch the tail end of a dream that goes as follows:

> . . . The movie has already started and some guy is talking about being an actor and he has a certain pair of shoes and we start to try and get the name of the shoes so we guess we can be an actor. The shoes have a particular sole on them and we try to find out what it is.

Do we take this dream literally? We might. We might say to ourself, yes, perhaps being an actor would be fun. Still, we are not buying air tickets for Hollywood. It might just be that as a sort of adjunct to our present life, acting might have a place.

The thing to keep in mind, whatever we dream—as we work on our particular goal—is how does it help us to KEEP OURSELF FROM SMOKING. If acting is some viable input in the equation, then it needs serious consideration. If we cannot handle the idea right now, then let it go.

Not everything can be handled equally. Possibly, not everything has to be considered, but we each have to find our way in this work. One man's recipe for corn bread might be another man's recipe for bane.

DAY FORTY-TWO—SUNDAY

For becoming more and more aware (through love) of HOW TO KEEP MYSELF FROM SMOKING—

Today I will work on my *Higher Thinking Center* with material from the following dreams:

> Something about being at a bank and wanting to renew our Master Card—it has expired—and being told the person who does that isn't in. We begin to get quite indignant in our mind about it. But we don't seem to make a big issue of it. . . . We seem to be somewhere else—about to buy something—and again wondering if they have a way we can renew our Master Card and use it. . . . We seem to be at a Hebrew lesson and using our Master Card or about to use it.

It does seem curious how for the last several nights there has been some sort of concern about 'credit'—other people's and our own. Our dream last night or this morning is similar; the slight difference is encouraging: From trying to renew the card at the beginning, to wondering about using it at the middle, we seem to wind up using it at the end.

. . . All of us need to hope that from here on, we shall receive some very practical suggestions that will truly allow us to KEEP OURSELF FROM SMOKING. But with dreams, we never have a guarantee. We may have new obstacles and new guideposts and the suggestions may not be as clear as we would like. Nevertheless, let us always try to remember that we are safe. It is only our best that dreams have in mind, provided we are open to what they are saying. We cannot have things, sometimes, the way we may have grown accustomed to having them. Sometimes, we have to make a choice between going it the old way, with all the bruises that we get, or trying to do it a different way, where there also may be bruises, but 'of independence.'

Another dream that we may record might go something like the following:

> There is also some dream with an old friend in it—and we can't recall what happens—though it seems time is running out but there is no panic.

With just one week left on our journey, time IS running out. But hopefully, that will be a good thing: by then we ought to be able to KEEP OURSELF FROM SMOKING.

DAY FORTY-THREE—MONDAY

For becoming more and more aware (through love) of HOW TO KEEP MYSELF FROM SMOKING—

Today I will work on my *Instinctive Center* with material from the following dreams:

Often our dreams may be painting some kind of picture of us that is just not the way we are, or so we think. We may find ourself going over a dream and there just may not be anything to experience except a kind of numbness. What can we do? After all, we are on our last week and we look in vain for any definite images about HOW TO KEEP OURSELF FROM SMOKING.

We may be selling a dream's power short. The very lack of 'an experience from the dream' may signal some sort of resistance that we are having about HOW TO KEEP OURSELF FROM SMOKING. If we persist, we may suddenly see that really things are not as bad as they seem. We have made some sort of progress. It may only come at the last dream or so, after we have been through a kind of frustrating time with the first one or two.

Let us look at a couple of uncomplimentary dreams that we may have during last night or early this morning:

> It seems we are at some party—perhaps some sort of self-awareness group—and then some parents pick up a daughter and we say goodbye to them as they are settling in the car—calling them 'folks.' The party has gone from meeting to after-meeting and people are now standing

> around the men's room—and we need to go—but we go outside instead—it is already light—we think of taking a long walk but it is already daylight. We have on a suit coat but are naked below.

After that dream, we may experience something like the following:

> There is a dream showing an old school chum having a list of dreams on a very beautiful brown satin vellum card—and one thing is the Roger Award for something. Then it seems we are with some other guys from high school and then we see another school chum and some girl and she's talking about some place where she wants to be. Then he seems to take some old papers and read them. Then we're driving someone else's new Jeep and it's hard to drive. We seem to have trouble stopping—and handling it. But we keep ourself as awake as we can. Then we seem to hit an area where all the lights go off—including the Jeep's. Then we get them on shortly—but one of the passengers says in the meantime they have done something. We can't even recall it.

Now after working on these two dreams, which really did not give us any kind of lasting experience—and left us feeling dismayed—perhaps we have the following two short dreams that seem to tell a different story:

> There is something about having got a truck lined up for delivery which seems to make us feel really quite happy.
>
> Also, something about maybe two trucks will be able to deliver.

So what can we say with all of this material on our plate? We can only say that we should never despair with our dreams. A link exists between them and us and we need to hammer away at the gap until after inches of steadfast planking we bring ourself closer to what they are about.

What is the key? Perhaps it is only never to give up, always to feel that there is SOMETHING THERE that we only have to work at for it to be realized and made useful for our lives. As to HOW TO KEEP OURSELF FROM SMOKING, perhaps we just have to go through many inappropriate images and self-embarrassing roles before we are ready to get a 'truck or two lined up for delivery.'

DAY FORTY-FOUR—TUESDAY

For becoming more and more aware (through love) of HOW TO KEEP MYSELF FROM SMOKING—

Today I will work on my *Sexual Center* with material from the following dreams:

As we continue recording our dreams every night, it may sometimes happen that instead of getting few dreams to write about, we find ourself with four dreams and maybe three of them are quite long. We cannot just spend the day on dreams and there is really nothing to do but do the best we can. Often out of all the words we have recorded it almost seems as if we say nothing much. It is always when we have that sort of reaction that we have to smile and try to realize that probably the case is just the opposite. What we are reading and thinking the dreams say, is probably not quite what they are saying. We can probably help ourself by trying to focus as much as we can on our goal—becoming aware of HOW TO KEEP OURSELVES FROM SMOKING—and on our particular center, here, the *Sexual Center.*

We should not take seriously our 'sense' that the words are 'going over our head' or not registering in our heart. We really do not know. The chemistry of dreams is a mystery and the words and scenes and settings may have a kind of meaning that is really not understood by us very well. At least not on our so-called conscious level.

Nevertheless, let us try to tell ourself that we are like an audience listening to a piece of modern music for the first time. A lot of us will feel there is little coherence. Yet forty years go by and another audience hearing the same piece of music really understands or relates to it. Our dreams are like the first hearing. Since they are 'ours' we cannot afford to wait forty years. We need to work hard on them now. THEN, perhaps, if we are still around in forty years, we will have a greater capacity for receiving dreams and perhaps even be more developed in significant ways.

Let us look at one dream that we may have, and try as we look at it to see if we can connect anything with our goal of HOW TO KEEP OURSELF FROM SMOKING:

> We dream about being at some country club with an old friend and we're talking with some guy and it turns out his dad has a big company like someone we've long heard about and we talk with his dad who seems to get tearful over something—and we say he's crying because he doesn't have enough money—or something like that. It may have been about kids or being moved, about family or something. And our old friend asks the father how the son is—and then adds: 'Because the son seems to be interested in working for (his) company.' The father seems agreeable—and our old friend assures him he'll have food on the table. As we watch our old friend eat—we see him bringing a lot of food to his mouth—then removing a lot of it. Then later we seem to be outside trying to get a ride with the son—but we don't seem to recall what he looks like or what to look for in the way of cars.

Is there not a kind of provocative mystery in all of this? Do we not have some sort of 'obligation' to stay with this sort of thing as long as we can?

There is an initiation process here, we believe. We can easily scoff at the whole thing and cast it aside, or we can accept the difficulty of the task and work as creatively (and stubbornly) as we can.

Along with the previously recorded dream, perhaps we have one similar to the following:

> There is something about evidence—how it can change or become one thing

> at one point and another at another point. We think our old friend is in on this too.

Here we cannot help wondering if the evidence against smoking that we have long been familiar with is not subtly changing its 'shape' and becoming something else—something that will impel us in some harmonious way to KEEP OURSELF FROM SMOKING.

DAY FORTY-FIVE—WEDNESDAY

For becoming more and more aware (through love) of HOW TO KEEP MYSELF FROM SMOKING—

Today I will work on my *Moving Center* with material from the following dreams:

What does it mean when we say that we are going to WORK ON our dreams? What is the WORK? We really cannot spell it out as easily as we would like. It concerns an effort that we make to deal with the material that we are given. Sometimes the work might be to 'try to believe' what is being said. Sometimes the work might be to 'try to do something suggested,' and perhaps more often than anything, the work might be just to sit quietly and proclaim what is being said in the dream. Often it is just to probe the words and phrases continuously, trying to get some sort of experience out of the material. Often, there may be nothing tangibly received or experienced. Yet sometimes, even when we think we have really not 'worked very productively,' we may have some kind of result. It may come as a kind of 'interesting or positive feeling.' We could not really define it to anyone, but something has moved within us because of the dream.

Such a dream might be the one we have on this night or early morning:

> We're driving along and as we approach an intersection a bus is in the middle sort of slowly making a turn and we can't tell whether to prepare in our mind to cross or wait—we can't see whether the light is green, red or what. As the bus finally crosses we see that the light is orange and we move ahead, but then it turns red and there we are still crossing on red. There are cars ahead and it seems a police car is stopped and is backing up to us or eventually does and we are concerned about getting a ticket. But nothing happens, though we soon find ourself at a filling station and are being lectured to by someone—as we brush our teeth. Then a face under a chef's hat appears and says hello—someone who apparently we have known from something before.

Why did we feel good about the dream? Perhaps the fellow under the chef's hat did the trick. He might be saying, "Remember me? Don't forget what has been said about food. Don't keep putting off what has been said."

Perhaps for us, and maybe others too, food is really a significant factor when it comes to learning how to KEEP OURSELF FROM SMOKING. We would not have thought so, but we have to reflect on the importance that it has played in our dreams during this journey of ours.

If we, in fact, are what we eat, then the sooner we eat differently than the way we have been eating, perhaps the sooner we can KEEP OURSELF FROM SMOKING. We may have been expecting something quite different and maybe there is more to it than food, but food seems to play a key role, at least according to the clues we have been receiving.

There is an old saying—"God wants us to relax and study things"—that might apply to this situation we are in: We are getting information—we might REACT and say 'NO WAY,' or we may feel FRUSTRATED or PUT UPON, and would like nothing more than to be done with the whole project. We have invested our time and our spirit and perhaps we would do far better in serving our best interests if we would just "relax and study things."

Perhaps for some of us, there is something other than food. Maybe food is not mentioned at all. Very well, whatever our information, let us try to approach it in the same spirit. Let us try to relax and study it—and see where it takes us.

DAY FORTY-SIX—THURSDAY

For becoming more and more aware (through love) of HOW TO KEEP MYSELF FROM SMOKING—

Today I will work on my *Emotional Center* with material from the following dreams:

The birth of an idea within us may occur so gradually that before we know it is there, we find ourself convinced that we must simply do what we have been nurturing. There is no sudden burst of awareness as much as a new sense of our responsibility. One minute we may be one way, and the next, we are another new way. So it might be as we get toward the end of this journey of HOW TO KEEP OURSELF FROM SMOKING. Perhaps we have a dream similar to the following:

> There is something about having a big school bus—and parking it on a street where we think some health-conscious relatives live. We may even have them pick us up and tell them we would be parking it where they live. We notice some interior designing or decoration on the second floor, when we are driving to where they live.

Something here makes us feel we are a bit different. Health IS becoming an issue. Words are no longer all we need, there is a new idea about responsibility.

Somehow, during all this, we are reminded of an old phrase we heard somewhere: "The healthier is better than the easier"—which we begin to understand a little better than we used to. What does it mean for us now? Only that we have to, in some gradual way, disturb our predilection for the life of ease. We cannot just 'go along' crediting ourselves for a stability that is harnessed to our smoking habit and driven by a kind of self-induced dependence on tobacco. It just will not wash any more (for us). We have to be committed to a different sort of responsibility. And along with the preceding dream, perhaps we have the following:

> Something about having a Party four months from now.

The idea of a party in the midst of all the serious things we have been addressing seems like a good sign for us. Whether it is a party of celebration (WE HAVE BEEN ABLE TO KEEP OURSELF FROM SMOKING FOR SO LONG . . .) or a party celebrating some new awareness of appreciation (SINCE WE HAVE BEEN KEEPING OURSELF FROM SMOKING, we have been so grateful for the scent of flowers, the ways we experience air, etc.) we really do not know. Nevertheless, a party sounds like a good idea, a good result after what we have been involved with.

And lastly, perhaps we have a dream like this one:

> We see an employee through our shop window sitting at a table maybe looking at some plans and we want to get him started on something.

AT LAST, we really are going to KEEP OURSELF FROM SMOKING. We really do want to get started on something and we really feel we can.

DAY FORTY-SEVEN—FRIDAY

For becoming more and more aware (through love) of HOW TO KEEP MYSELF FROM SMOKING—

Today I will work on my *Thinking Center* with material from the following dreams:

Occasionally we may have a dream that is outright pornographic. We are struck with the fact that we are involved without any sort of remorse. How can this be? The energy that we experience may not be all that bad for us. Rather than cast the dream aside, and act as if it 'must be a mistake,' perhaps we should look at it, particularly in the light of our desire to learn HOW TO KEEP OURSELF FROM SMOKING, and, in this case, to work on our *Thinking Center*.

If we take a dream that outwardly seems quite inappropriate for us, and try to link it with our two goals, we may find something that is quite beneficial for us. At the risk of offending some, we would like to see if we can explain this process in a way that might help us generate a certain energy toward our goal without upsetting our 'particular outward morality.'

Perhaps we have a dream on this night or early morning that goes as follows:

> We're in some condo and go to a locker room—shower area—where we're standing naked and some girl appears and apparently she needs to get something around where we are standing—and we kind of go around each other trying to avoid bumping into each other's pubic areas. She jokes that we're trying to impregnate her. Then we seem to bring her close to us and we start holding her tight little butt and we're sort of bumping each other.

Now on the face of this, we are into nothing more nor less than unadulterated smut. Perhaps we are, but dreams are not as concerned with what we think we should be as with what will perhaps HELP US TO BE. For most of us, this sort of dream is a shock to our 'modesty.' It gets our attention, if nothing else.

We want to use the energy in this dream to help us with our goal—particularly HOW TO KEEP OURSELF FROM SMOKING.

If we go back to the dream, and try to 'run through it,' we find that there is a real jolt of energy where we are 'holding her tight little butt.' Now if we link that with our desire to become aware of HOW TO KEEP OUR-

SELF FROM SMOKING, we find a kind of determination to achieve that goal above any sexual profligacy. Perhaps the energy of sex CAN be used for something more than sex. There is a legitimate way of fusing one kind of energy (in a dream) with something we want to achieve in real life.

Undoubtedly there is an area here, where 'inner fantasy' could become a problem, but if we simply take what has been given 'in a dream' and work with it, without trying to induce side issues into the process, we may find something that we really can use and benefit from.

. . . We are going to be parting company in a few days. By this time we should be close to saying to ourself: I AM KEEPING MYSELF FROM SMOKING, I CAN KEEP MYSELF FROM SMOKING, I AM ABLE TO KEEP MYSELF FROM SMOKING.

We may have a dream similar to the following:

> It seems as if someone says we really looked good last night.

We need to keep up with our 'wisdom cards' and try to reflect on those things that can give us reinforcement as we KEEP OURSELF FROM SMOKING. We have only a few more days and for some of us there might be more activities in our daily life than we can manage without lessening our concentration on our dreams. If that happens, so be it. We can try to do only as much as we are able and if we do find a lessening of concentration, perhaps it simply shows that we have really done enough by this point. We may not need much more of this journey.

For those of us who really have not seen enough, perhaps the next few nights will tell it all. This work can be very subtle in its effect on us. We may not really think we are ready to KEEP OURSELF FROM SMOKING, but some little incident might reveal that we are ready, that we can begin.

DAY FORTY-EIGHT—SATURDAY

For becoming more and more aware (through love) of HOW TO KEEP MYSELF FROM SMOKING—

Today I will work on my *Higher Emotional Center* with material from the following dreams:

There is an interesting aspect of dreams that we have touched on before, but it seems that we need to touch on it again. It is an aspect that we might call 'verification of our effort,' or 'a positive reinforcement of what we have attempted'—and it works for all of us as it works for one.

It might be at this point in our journey that we dream something which compliments us on what we have been attempting. Perhaps we have begun to KEEP OURSELF FROM SMOKING, and we are doing it with 'lack of full confidence in ourself.' True, we feel we are okay, but how pleasant it would be to receive some unexpected good words from a dream.

In an effort merely to show how it might be for someone in our shoes, we reluctantly reproduce the following dream:

> An image of someone going up to top of steps—having entertained or something and we are behind him and when he gets to top we say: 'Well done.' Not exclamatorily—sort of softly but sincerely.

Again, on this night or early morning, we receive the following dream:

> We also hear one of our near-and-dear ones talking to another near-and-dear one about the book and one tells the other it has some fellow-sufferers in mind, positive thinking, etc. and one of them says: "No one is too stupid not to understand this book."

And now, let us return to the remainder of our journey, the last two nights and two days, perhaps the most important part for some of us . . .

DAY FORTY-NINE—SUNDAY

For becoming more and more aware (through love) of HOW TO KEEP MYSELF FROM SMOKING—

Today I will work on my *Higher Thinking Center* with material from the following dreams:

We have reached the end of our journey. All who have stuck it out are to be congratulated. It has probably been next to impossible to be 'true all the way,' but there has been tremendous effort and a concentrated ambition and that is often enough, to achieve what we need to achieve. At any rate, the time has come to say goodbye or close to it. We have the past night's dreams and early morning dreams to discuss and then we will celebrate our freedom, which hopefully we either have or are close to having, with the FIFTIETH NIGHT AND DAY. So let us look at our dreams last night or early this morning and try to see what we have.

Those of us who have already committed ourselves to KEEPING OURSELF FROM SMOKING may now be having dreams that reflect a concern about 'not making it.' That is probably normal, since there is always a residue of doubt, whatever we do. The only thing is to bring it into the light of day, smile at it, as if it were a small child coming into the bedroom after having moved to a new house, and comfort it with an understanding word. We are always going to have such moments, even if we live to be a hundred. There are aspects of ourself that are always going to need comforting. And that is all they need. They do not have to dictate a new direction, but they are entitled to some concerned attention.

The following is a dream that we might have:

> There is some concern on our part that one of our cars will break down and we'll need to get another one and we tell this to one near-and-dear-to-us who seems to be slightly overwhelmed by us buying another car. We have just got several. We then sort of say, perhaps we'll just drive it until it breaks down. Then get another one.

Can we see how that connects with our KEEPING OURSELF FROM SMOKING? Isn't there a fear that perhaps the new habit—KEEPING OURSELF FROM SMOKING—might break down? What do we do then? Well, it is a 'new habit,' why should it break down so quickly? We are just using it. We do not need to reinforce it with something else yet. Time will take care of what we do, if our present way of KEEPING OURSELF

FROM SMOKING breaks down. Let us just focus on 'operating it correctly' for now. Perhaps when it is time for something else, we will know what to do.

Perhaps we have a dream like the following one on this night or early morning:

> We're someplace and happen to see a deceased influential person come in with a kid. He looks terrible, but tries to identify with us. Then someone else also tries —showing us he buttons his middle shirt button (the way we do our jacket).

Here again, perhaps, influences are calling upon us that want to 'bring us back to where we were.' It is natural, and all we can do is recognize what they are and avoid them. As we have said before, if we possibly can or if we can possibly remember to remind ourself—we should love things as we also find ourself reacting against them. Again, we might have another sort of 'disturbing dream' that goes as follows:

> It also seems as if we are on some sort of lounge chair and someone comes along and tries to tip us or turn it.

There is always going to be some sort of 'opposition'—it is part of the human contract—and the best we can hope for is a 'managed opposition'—one that might disturb us but never overcome us.

So let us now turn our thoughts to managed freedom from the habit of smoking. Let us celebrate, after FORTY-NINE DAYS OF BONDAGE, the FIFTIETH ONE THAT PROCLAIMS OUR FREEDOM.

DAY FIFTY—MONDAY
THE JUBILEE

For becoming more and more aware (through love) of HOW TO KEEP MYSELF FROM SMOKING—

Today—THE JUBILEE—I will work on my *Instinctive Center* with material from the following dreams:

Well, perhaps we should kick back and relax and enjoy our freedom from smoking—whether it is actual or symbolic. We have been in bondage for so many years. Now at least we know it and have either taken steps TO KEEP OURSELF FROM SMOKING, or hopefully, intend to do so very soon. At such a time of celebration what can we do? Perhaps our dreams last night show the sort of thing that is appropriate:

> It seems we or someone are singing some song, making fun of some defense man—we reflect how we don't seem to have songs today about the defense people.

Though we are celebrating, thinking about this dream might be fun, for it does seem to talk about something that we do not seem to do. Maybe it would help if we did: Sing about the defense people. Who are they? Perhaps we can only hazard a guess.

When we started on this journey, we had a dream that seemed to reflect 'resistance' to the idea of KEEPING OURSELF FROM SMOKING. That was one of the defense people. There must be a ton of them running around inside us, always voicing concern about something that we might have concluded we should do, but what do they do? They say all the reasons why it will not work. So, in a moment of victory, perhaps it is fitting to sing a song making fun of 'some defense man'—the one who said in some way that we could not pull off this idea of KEEPING OURSELF FROM SMOKING. Like a troubadour of old, perhaps each of us can compose a song deriding this defense man, letting him know in a happy form, that we did it, we overcame the opposition, and now we are free of him.

Sometimes, during a celebration of this nature, people have a tendency to 'probe' into their successful venture and try to find out more than perhaps they should. There is always a tendency to want to get to the bottom of some phenomenon such as HOW DID I START KEEPING MYSELF FROM SMOKING. Perhaps against this mental framework, we might have the following dream on our Jubilee night or early morning:

> We are with some guy in a classy part of town—we think a sort of snobbish sort—and we get out an excavator and are going to try to do something with it—but where we want to go is really rough—one area is quite steep and the other is enclosed with a fence. Finally we seem to reach a point where we say—'Let's just leave things as they are'—and are going to put the excavator back where we found it. There just isn't anything to do . . . The guy we are with has found a cat but comments now he can't find it. Then we happen to be on top of a roof—where a grate is and another cat starts

> throwing a ball through it to another cat below who throws it back and they get into a real game of catch. It is 'incredible' seeing them throw this ball back and forth.

May we (all) find "our cats," enjoy "their game of catch," and KEEP OURSELVES FROM SMOKING!

Printed in the United States
2001